The Hot Mom's Handbook

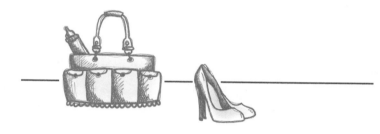

The Hot Mom's
HANDBOOK

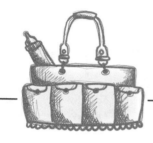

BY
JESSICA DENAY

wm

WILLIAM MORROW
An Imprint of HarperCollins*Publishers*

This book is written as a source of information only. The information contained in this book should by no means be considered as a substitute for the advice, decisions, or judgment of the reader's physician or other professional advisor.

All efforts have been made to ensure the accuracy of the information contained in this book as of the date published. The author and the publisher expressly disclaim responsibility for any adverse effects arising from the use or application of the information contained herein.

FIRST EDITION

Designed by Diahann Sturge

Library of Congress Cataloging-in-Publication Data is available upon request.

ISBN 978-0-06-178737-9

11 12 13 14 15 OV/RRD 10 9 8 7 6 5 4 3 2 1

This book belongs to Hot Mom:

_____

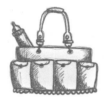

For my mom:
For teaching me to always keep a sense of humor, for indulging my visions, and for never putting a ceiling on my sky

For my son, Gabriel:
For opening up a new dimension of love in my heart and being

Contents

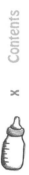

Big Fat o' Disclaimer

I have been called a mother's lifestyle expert, but let me make it clear that I am *not* an expert at being a mom—no one is and no one can be, whether she has twenty-seven kids or has been parenting for 150-plus years. We are all learning day by day. Each child is different; each circumstance is different. Like you, I am doing the best I can every day, making choices—some good ones, some I wish I could do over. Parenting is filled with mistakes. It's about learning from our mistakes and learning from others who have been through similar circumstances. No one is perfect. That is not what this book is about. It's not going to groom you to be the perfect Stepford mom, and it's not going to scare you silly with all the dangers in the world. It's filled with straight-up, simple, and practical advice and tons of great products to make your post-baby life easier and more fun. Everything has been sourced for you. All of the products chosen have been Hot Moms Club tested and approved. No companies have paid for their products to be included in this book. I and the Hot Moms Club team have tried hundreds of products throughout the years and are privy to the latest and newest on the market, and I am sharing our favorites with you.

I am also NOT a doctor, nor do I play one on TV. Always,

always, always check with your physician before doing anything new. This book is a guide full of great suggestions, but it should never take the place of your doctor's advice.

Okay, now that we have gotten that cleared up, on to the book!

Preface

(AKA the important backstory as to why
I wrote this book and what you can expect)

*I'd like to be the ideal mother,
but I'm too busy raising my kids.*
—Unknown

There are so many different parenting styles and parenting circumstances, and there are a bazillion ways to be a great mom. My hope is that there is something in this book everyone can connect to, be it a story, perspective, idea, or quotation. I've made mistakes as a parent, and luckily you will be able to learn from them. Like you, all I can do is use what I learn to be the best mom I can be today, tomorrow, and the days that follow. Some days I get an A, and, well, other times . . . let's just say it's not always easy to bridge the gap between knowing things and applying them. But being a Hot Mom is not about being perfect or doing it all; that would be impossible—not to mention boring. Being a Hot Mom is finding balance and happiness in your life so that your child will have a chance at balance and happiness in hers or his. It's about doing your best in each moment and, most importantly, having fun and enjoying the ride, starting right now.

This book is filled with the experiences of fascinating mothers I have met through the Hot Moms Club. I have written it in "bite size" portions. I get it: we moms are busy. My goal was to keep it simple so you can read it when you get a free minute here and there, be it waiting for the school bell to ring or soccer practice to let out.

So what is a Hot Mom, anyway? A Hot Mom is a woman who is confident and empowered. It doesn't matter what age you are, what shape or size, EVERY mom can be a Hot Mom! It's a choice. It's an attitude and a way of being. It's knowing that you are not the best mom unless you are the best YOU.

My friend Joy and I started the Hot Moms Club six years ago because we wanted to create a website and network that spoke to moms as women, not just as parents. (Believe it or not, there was nothing like it back then. Boy, have things evolved!)

At the Hot Moms Club we believe motherhood gives us depth, compassion, and a level of love and awareness so heartfelt it is indescribable. When our children are born, so is this other person, a mom—this ever-caring, protective, beck-and-call being. We now have these babies who came to us, or they came through us, and we help mold them, teach them, and yet each is his or her own person; they are entities of their own with their own destinies and connections to the world. It's important that while we help shape and nurture our children's world we each keep nurturing and creating our own spirit. A Hot Mom knows the importance of keeping the balance between her true self and her self as a mother. A Hot Mom radiates this confidence. A

Hot Mom loves herself and her family but doesn't get consumed by the madness of motherhood. Hot Moms know how to balance *their* needs and the needs of their families.

There is a Hot Mom inside of every mom. This book will give you all the tools to break her loose. The goal of this book is to help you connect or reconnect to your true self and to encourage you NOT to abandon your identity but rather to embrace it and become a Hot Mom. After all, a Hot Mom is a BETTER mom! A Hot Mom is a BETTER lover! A Hot Mom is a BETTER friend!

Hot: *(adj) Arousing intense excitement.*

Moms: *(n, pl) Women who nurture children.*

Club: *(n) A group organized for a common purpose.*

This book is an updated version of the original published in 2005. They say we teach best what we most need to learn, and I believe that was true with the earlier edition. I am in a much different place now from when I wrote this book six years ago. The state of motherhood has been successfully redefined. This is evident when I reread my original preface. Those are the words of a young mom searching, feeling, and saying she was empowered but needing reinforcement to really believe it. I needed the network of moms I was building as much as they needed the Hot Moms Club. My son and I have grown leaps and bounds. My baby is now ten and almost as tall as me. Just like an exercise routine I have adopted and practiced, the tips and ideas I talk about in this book have become incorporated into my life—and they really work. I am living proof, as I feel empowered now, I am confident now, I feel genuinely happy and grateful. I have had the privilege of meeting some of the most interesting and well-known women and respected experts in parenting. I am excited to share what I have learned from them with you.

There are so many "mommy myths" out there. This book puts them to bed (of course, tucked in with a kiss) and proves that being a great mom and being sexy don't have to be mutually exclusive. It's time to move out of that comfortable rut. These chapters hold simple, blunt, to-the-point guidance for the body and soul that is GUARANTEED to transform any mom into a HOT MOM.

Foreword

By Lauren Holly

I was thirty-eight when I became a mom for the first time. (Older by many people's standards, younger by other's.) I now have three sons: Azer, George, and Henry. I became a mom at the right time for me. I knew that our relationship could be one of mutual enrichment, albeit a noisy one!

Instinctually, I keep them safe, nurture them, and prepare them for their future. I am a mom! But my boys do the same for me. Azer loves my traditions, and his memory of details is astounding. He loves the repetition that traditions bring, and I have the comfort of knowing I'll leave a legacy. He especially loves my silly traditions, like birthdays, which are always exciting, but I thought Mom's birthday should be exciting, too. No, I don't have hats and noisemakers, but I do have two cakes. The second cake is just for fun. The boys strip down and we have a cake fight. The first year this occurred in the dining room; we've since moved it outside! Mom's birthday has become a tradition we look forward to all year.

George loves beauty. He seems so proud when I dress up, and he loves to make anything a special occasion. We plan special dinners, when we all dress up and wear our "fancy" shoes. The way he looks at me stays with me for days.

Henry loves being silly, which is wonderful, as I love being silly, too. I love to blast the stereo and dance any way I want to. So does he. We often dance and dance until we're sweaty. It doesn't matter what stresses are going on in my day, crazy dancing melts them all away. All the boys join in, and a good night's sleep is all that's on the agenda!

Ultimately, children learn by example. They do what they see. My boys see that I take my job seriously and work very hard. They see that I take care of myself. I eat healthy foods, exercise, get plenty of sleep, and am loving and affectionate. I talk about things and listen to what is being said. Mommy and Daddy sometimes need private time, but my boys like their own private time, too. I make sure to love myself as well as my sons. My boys' self-esteem grows and grows as they learn to love themselves as well as others. Take what I know and apply it, and no matter what age you are, you too can be a Hot Mom!

LAUREN HOLLY is a film and TV actress best known for her roles in *Chicago Hope*, *Picket Fences*, and *NCIS*, as well as in the hit movie *Dumb and Dumber*, with Jim Carrey, to whom she was briefly married. Today Lauren is at her happiest. She has found the balance between career and motherhood. She is a happily married mom raising and enjoying her three adopted sons.

Special Sections You'll Find Throughout This Book

BABY ON A BUDGET

Let's face it: It's expensive to raise a child today. Everyone is looking for ways to save money. For this reason, I've included Baby on a Budget sections with practical, penny-pinching tips and ideas.

ECO-MINDED MAMA

It is never too early to make your little ones environmentally conscious and healthy. Thankfully, there are many great green options today in childrearing, from maternity and beyond. In each chapter of the book I have added eco-friendly or organic alternatives to minimize your baby's "carbon butt print" and to preserve your peace of mind.

DADS ARE THE NEW MOMS

Dads are more involved than ever in raising children. It is more socially accepted and more of an expectation today than it ever was before. Throughout the coming pages I share some creative ways to trick—I mean, *get dad engaged in* the process.

$TUFF TO DROOL OVER

The number of luxury baby items on the market (AKA the outrageously overpriced and completely overindulgent and unnecessary in everyway, yet fabulous) never ceases to amaze me. Just for fun, I have included some of my favorites in various categories sprinkled throughout the book. And for those who can afford them, I provide all of the purchasing information.

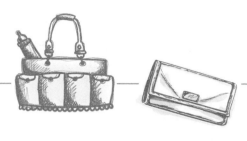

One

From BC (Before Child) to AD (After Delivery)

It's not easy being a mother.
If it were easy, fathers would do it.

—The Golden Girls

I wasn't always a Hot Mom. The Hot Moms Club was born out of my need to feel confident and bridge the gap between the person I was BC (before child) and the frazzled mother I had become.

As my son entered that crazy, wacky, "what the hell am I going to do with him?" toddler stage, it became harder and harder to juggle the latest trends, a social life, and the responsibilities of motherhood. Keeping my wardrobe current was the

Balance: (n)

1. *An even distribution of weight enabling someone or something to remain upright and steady.*
2. *Stability of one's mind or feelings.*
3. *A condition in which different elements are equal or in the correct proportions.*

least of my concerns; shaving not one but both legs in the shower became a luxury. Like so many moms do, I fell victim to convenience. I would roll out of bed, pile my hair into a ponytail, sniff and shuffle through the hamper, toss on the most comfy sweats that didn't look too dirty, and head to the park.

To my horror, I had come to fit the mom stereotype and all that went with it. My main focus and the point of my existence seemed to be my son's comfort and happiness. My day revolved around *Groundhog Day*–like errands and his activities. I lost myself in this routine. Where was that confident, fun-loving person I was BC? Did being a good mom mean that my spirit had to suffer? I was depressed. I thought, This isn't supposed to be *my* life! I was your classic overachiever from a good family and nice small town. My life was textbook until about age twenty-four. I got pregnant with a man I hadn't been dating very long. We got married and we got divorced. Here I was, to my shock and horror, twenty-five and a single mom. This wasn't supposed to happen to me . . . I was a "good girl." Where were my house, my husband, the dog, and the 2.5 kids? Adjusting to life as a single mom, I lost my confidence in everything that I was, *poof*—just like that. As much as I tried to keep my identity, the minute I mentioned to a date or to anyone else that I had a son, I fell victim to the mom stereotype and all that went with it. I was trying desperately to juggle the responsibilities and labels. How could I possibly be the best mom if I had so much inner frustration? Then it hit me: I couldn't blame people for holding tight to their image of what a mom should be when I clung so tight to the image of what my life should have been. I somehow believed that not having a husband or that "perfect" life was the reason I was stuck in the rut. It took me a long time to figure out but it wasn't my situation but my perception of it and my distorted perceptions of motherhood. I realized that if I wanted people to perceive me differently, I had to change the way I perceived myself and my life. I don't mean to get all Oprah on you, but the moment my attitude changed was the moment everything changed. You can't be the best mom when you are holding back your true self, when you are filled with self-doubt or frustration, when you are clinging tight to ideals, when you are doing things for everyone but yourself. It is crucial to foster you spirit and your passions. You have to stay true to your inner voice and indulge guilt-free in the little things that make you happy. It makes you a BETTER mom, it makes dads better dads, and your kids better kids.

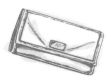

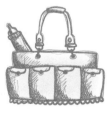

Before and After Kids

Before kids: You spend your time engaged in intellectually stimulating conversations with your colleagues.

After kids: Conversation? What's that? Nowadays, you spend your time trying to persuade your child to stop picking his nose in public.

Before kids: You slip lipstick and a credit card into a sleek handbag on your way out to the mall.

After kids: You stuff diapers, wipes, animal crackers, sippy cups, Band-Aids, coloring books, crayons, Thomas the Tank Engine, and a bottle of aspirin into your diaper bag on your way out to the playground.

Before kids: The kitchen floor is so clean you can eat off it.

After kids: You can eat off the kitchen floor because there's food all over it.

Before kids: You and your husband consistently enjoy hot sex.

After kids: You and your husband occasionally enjoy a hot meal.

Before kids: You coordinate the perfect outfit to wear for a night out dancing.
After kids: You grab something out of the laundry basket and pray that no one at the puppet show will notice the breast-milk stain.

Before kids: You save money to treat yourself to a Kate Spade handbag.
After kids: You save money to treat your son to a SpongeBob backpack.

Before kids: You dine on low-calorie, low-fat lunches at trendy new restaurants.
After kids: You wolf down someone's leftover pizza and cake at Chuck E. Cheese.

Before kids: You can easily finish a great book.
After kids: You're barely able to finish a simple thought.

> **Before kids:** Your idea of bliss is being with the love of your life.
>
> **After kids:** Your idea of bliss is tucking the love (or loves) of your life into bed each night.
>
> —Stephanie Blum,
> comedian, Hot Mom of three,
> and Hot Moms Club member

Motherhood can be overwhelming sometimes. We live in a society moving at lightning speed. We have too many obligations, and when someone wants something from us, even though we know we are overloaded we often take on more, pushing our own needs to the back burner. It's not easy. As moms, we have more responsibilities than ever, and we are functioning on less sleep, with pint-size people sabotaging our every move. I acknowledge—and live—firsthand the difficulties and challenges that have been the inevitable price of motherhood for everyone since the beginning of time. But with approximately four births every second around the world, take comfort in knowing that you are not alone. Now, this book isn't about complaining, it isn't about excuses, *it's about solutions*—practical, applicable solutions.

The only way you can achieve balance is if you take time for yourself. I am sure you are rolling your eyes about now, thinking, How can I make time for one more thing when I can barely get through what is on my plate now? The ironic and amazing thing is that once you start making time for yourself, claiming it no matter what, you will start feeling better about yourself, happier, more at peace, refreshed, and recharged, and your schedule and everything in it will be easier to deal with and fall into place. Trust me.

> Sometimes parents just need a break. To avoid feeling overwhelmed or overburdened, find time to replenish and nurture yourself. Take a five-minute walk, take a bath, or sneak into the bathroom to read a magazine so you can be alone for a few minutes. When your baby is napping, lie down and relax. When your child is at school, do something for yourself: Go to a bookstore and browse, get a massage, treat yourself to lunch or a movie, listen to self-improvement CDs, or take a coffee break. Twenty minutes soaking in the bathtub after the kids are asleep may not equal a week in Hawaii, but if it's all you have, make every moment count. Find the gratitude in every little moment that replenishes your soul and provides you with renewed energy to be the best mommy you can be.
>
> —Andrea Frank Henkart,
> Hot Mom of two, author,
> and motivational speaker

Busy Mom Obstacles

Obstacle #1: Finding—um, *making* the time

Solution: Claim time. It's that simple. As mothers, we are multitasking goddesses, and we do it all with a toddler strapped to our hip. If you decide that taking time for yourself each day or each week is a priority, you will make it happen. So just as you squeeze in that doctor's appointment or you schedule a nanny for work, schedule "you time." If it means the dishes are still in the sink, so be it. Start with ten to fifteen minutes each day, make it happen, then work your way to a full hour once a week. Maybe it's a yoga class, a hike, a manicure, or just sitting in your backyard in the sun—something little each day and week that's all yours.

I remember during the summers growing up, after playing and swimming all morning, my mom would enforce quiet time for one hour in our rooms after lunch. We used to complain and ask, Why, why? My mom would say, "You need to digest your food and relax." I remember lying in my bed waiting desperately for that time to be up so we could go back outside and play and swim again. As I got older, my mom would let me come into her room with her. During this hour, she would watch her soap opera (*All My Children*) and fold clothes or iron. I didn't realize it then, but that was her way of claiming that hour each day for herself. It was her time. Granted, she was still being productive, but it was peaceful and it was hers. Had I realized then how important that was for her, I wouldn't have given her such a hard time. Sorry, Mom.

> When my son was nearing the age of no more naps, I felt anxious about losing my break in the day to make phone calls or take a much-needed rest. Rather than giving this time up, I told my son we would now be having "quiet time." He now spends one hour midday in his room flipping through his favorite books, listening to stories on CD, or quietly playing. I now have a regular time I can count on to myself, and he has learned the discipline to wait until his special kitchen timer dings before he can come out of his room and resume the day. We both look forward to this midday break. Everyone needs some down time.
>
> —Kimberle Gamble,
> cofounder of NurturedPath.com

Obstacle #2: Finding someone to watch the kids

Solution: Relatives. If you've got 'em close by, you are truly lucky. (Mine are three thousand miles away.) Don't take them for granted for a second. Lean on them, but make sure you show your appreciation with notes and cards from you and the kids after they babysit. Not only will it make them feel appreciated, it will strengthen their desire to help. (Kids love decorating cards and sending them in the mail. If you have a little baby, you can write the note from their imagined perspective and stamp it with a hand or footprint.)

And then there's the excuse, "I don't have anyone I can trust."

I get it: The recurring nightmares of some teenage girl texting her newest crush while Junior eats junk food all night have you a bit apprehensive. But ask friends, coworkers, and neighbors for referrals and find a sitter you like. Start having him or her come while you are home to get the kids adjusted; this will enable you to get some things done around the house while they are getting to know each other. Always have a great sitter or two up your sleeve for last-minute invites, etc.

Sittercity.com is a great resource. You pop in your zip code and they will connect you to prescreened girls in your area that fit your needs and your budget.

Another solution: Leave the kids with your hubby. It is really good for dads to have this time alone with the kids. When kids are with both parents, they naturally defer to Mom. If Dad watches the kids more often, they will be more likely come to him for nurturing and problem-solving. It is a great way for them to bond.

BABY ON A BUDGET

Start a babysitting co-op. Gather a group of parents with kids in the same age range as your child or children, people you trust and kids you wouldn't mind watching yourself. Create a currency; for example, each family starts with ten tokens, each representing one hour of babysitting time. If you need a babysitter for two hours while you go to a class or dinner, you give two tokens to the person or couple watching the kids. The only way you can get more hours or time is by getting more tokens, meaning you need to babysit. This keeps things fair and balanced, so no one feels taken advantage of.

$TUFF TO DROOL OVER

Westside Nannies is the premier nanny service out of Beverly Hills that many celebrities use. Prescreened and carefully selected, full-time nannies typically earn salaries ranging from $800 to $2,000 a week, or $40 an hour. Be prepared to also provide two weeks' vacation, health insurance, a car, and cell phone—not to mention the $2,500 to $4,500 placement fee for the agency.

Let dads help, and let them do it their way. This teaches our children that not everyone does things the same way, and it also builds confidence in the dads. Dads are quite capable if you let them share in the work, and this makes things so much easier when you need a girls' night out or a weekend away. When I leave for a weekend away I don't cook meals ahead of time, I don't make lists of thing he can do with the kids, and if I don't make it to the grocery store I don't worry. He can take the kids to the store, he can feed them and get them dressed, and he can plan his own day with them. When I get home he is usually more appreciative of me, and I am well rested and more appreciative of him!

—Justine Corey-Whitehead,
Hot Mom of two

DADS ARE THE NEW MOMS

Some guys are just natural with kids; others are a little nervous and it takes time to build their confidence. Boot Camp for New Dads (BootCampForNewDads.org) has classes all over the country. It has been described as a nursery in a locker room, with no women over two feet tall allowed. It's men teaching other men the ropes. Dads learn how to change diapers, soothe a crying infant, and get really comfortable with their little ones.

Obstacle #3: Guilt

Solution: Lose the guilt. As the mom, you are the nucleus of the family; your attitude sets the tone for everyone. Making time for yourself and your needs makes you a better mom. You need time to refresh and recharge. Remember, you are not the best mom unless you are the best YOU! Think of it as a balloon: You need to release and let a little air out once in a while. If it fills too much, it will pop. What benefit are you to your kids if you are on the verge of a breakdown or frazzled all the time? And what example are you setting? When you are balanced and doing things for yourself and your child spills grape juice on the carpet, you are less likely to freak out. You will be more calm, get it cleaned up, tell them it was an accident and to be more careful next time. But if you are spread too thin and your child accidentally spills grape juice on the carpet, you are more likely to snap and overreact. Your family deserves to have you at your happiest and your best. Creating harmony is crucial in your home for the well-being of your children. Taking time for yourself is a great gift you can give your family. Preserving your sanity is in their best interest, too, and something they will jump to support. So get over it—lose the guilt!

Kids Need a Break from Us, Too

There are few things that can make your heart ache like a two-year-old bear-hugging your shins sobbing, "Mommy, don't leave!" while you go out to enjoy a mediocre movie. But you deserve a life. Be confident, breathe deeply, and relax. Remember, kids, just like animals, can sense fear, and even very young children can sense a parent's anxiety. If you act nervous about leaving your little one with a sitter, they will pick up on it and become fearful and panicky. Make sure to prepare them all day or even a few days in advance.

Be sure to say good-bye when you leave and promise to kiss them when you get home. Do not try to avoid confrontation by dashing out the door while your little one is distracted playing a game of Chutes and Ladders; you are courting disaster and breeding a child that will never be sure when you are going to dart off, which will make him cling more, not less. Now, if you feel that your child takes a while to adjust to new people, have your sitter come over a few times while you are home and let them play while you do housework. I promise you, your children will survive a night without you, and might even enjoy it!

Growing up, I used to love when my parents went out because that meant Meghan was going to watch us. We LOVED Meghan. As a treat, my parents would order a pizza or buy TV dinners (I know) for the nights she came over. She let us stay up late and we played lots of games. It was so much fun. I learned early on that my parents always came back; it's good for kids to get a little independence and time away from you as well. Make it special for them. Give them a certain treat when sitters come so that they start to associate your date night or yoga class with something fun for them, too. It can be a win-win if you position it right.

Taking time for yourself each week or each day is a good exercise in letting go for both you and your baby.

Oxygen

When I used to sit on an airplane, waiting for takeoff, I was always surprised and frankly horrified as the flight attendant presented her canned speech, while she pointed to the exits with arms moving in cheerleader-like precision, explaining how we could save ourselves if the plane were to fall from the sky.

What horrified me was not the thought of free falling from the sky, but rather the instructions given to mothers, that in case of a drop in cabin pressure they were to put the oxygen masks on themselves first. Then and only then were they to put the masks on their children. It seemed so wrong, so cold and so selfish—really bad.

Then I had a baby. The baby grew into a child. I discovered that extreme mothering could lead to oxygen deprivation for the mother. Devoting every moment of every day to fulfilling my child's slightest needs, wants, and whims became not only exhausting but also caused me oxygen starvation. I couldn't breathe. One inspired day I came up for oxygen. I signed up for a watercolor class, two hours every Thursday night. One night a week of being unequivocally, self-lovingly me. Not a mother, not an employee, not anybody's girlfriend, just me.

Ahh . . . the oxygen that came pouring through. That pure, clean, fresh oxygen allowed me to breathe, deeply. As I began to breath deeper I noticed my son was breathing deeper, too, as was my boyfriend, and, it seemed, everyone around me.

I now take an oxygen break regularly, without guilt or a second thought, happy that in doing so I am showing my son and everyone who used to depend on me how to take their own oxygen and breathe, deeply.

—Carmen Richardson Rutlen,
from *Dancing Naked . . . In Fuzzy Red Slippers*

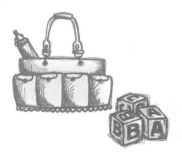

Who Needs Who?
The Industrial Strength Umbilical Cord

Let us start by admitting that we totally get it. One look at your sweet little heavenly creation and even the most indulgent woman withers away to nothing. It makes biological sense: nature looking out for its young. But at some point following infancy, a healthy mother is supposed to "cut the apron strings" and let little Landon fend for himself a bit. Some mothers are able to do this with ease. Maybe adopting an "if-it-don't-kill-'em" attitude does not work for you. But don't be a Stay-at-Home Martyr, either. Instead of shoving your little birdie from the nest, you would rather hand-stitch a giant double parachute and slowly cascade to the ground with your eaglet in tow. You may feel you have done the right thing by protecting your child, cushioning his fall, and staying by his side. Sadly, this little bird will not understand the principles of gravity or the importance of wing muscle development when he grows up. He will expect a homemade butt pillow at every bump in the road, and since Mom simply can't be there to scoop him up (as much as she would love to be), he'll be left to flounder his way through adulthood. You may not believe that you can actually care too much or do too much; maybe you think it is perfectly normal that your nine-year-old has never actually brushed his own teeth, or your six-year-old hyperventilates when you leave the room. Kids must learn to self-soothe. Never learning to cope with life's obstacles leads to the painful inability to function in the real world. Resentment will continually resurface (resentment toward everyone's favorite target (Mom)) every time Junior gets fired, dumped, or denied. So if you rush to your child when she so much as hiccups, you are teaching her that everything is catastrophic and warrants absolute hysteria. What's the result a child who falls apart at the sight of a hangnail?

—Joanne Kimes and Jennifer Worley, authors of *The Stay-At-Home Martyr*

Perfect: (adj) Entirely without faults or flaws.

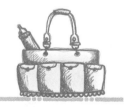

There is no way to be a perfect mother, and a million ways to be a good one.
—Jill Churchill

Step Away from the June Cleaver Ideal

I think part of our guilt as mothers centers on our desire to be perfect or be the best we can be. But being a martyr doesn't make you the best; it makes you a victim and it keeps you exhausted. We need to set an example, but remember, neither your kids nor anyone else expects you to be perfect. Aiming for perfection will only stress you out. It's okay to feel frustrated and overwhelmed; that is part of the price of admission of being a mom, and the more kids you have, the more demanding your schedule. Go easy on yourself, and remember: No mom is perfect, not one. Not June Cleaver, Carol Brady, not even Angelina or Jennifer Garner. They may seem perfect, toting their toddlers with glowing skin and ease . . . but every mother has stress, and flaws; some are just better at hiding it. Don't compare yourself to other moms in the carpool lane or at Gymboree, and especially don't compare yourself to celebrity moms. They have a team of people (chefs, assistants, stylists, nannies) helping them look fabulous and manage their busy schedules. Having worked with dozens of top-tier celebrity parents, I can assure you, they have the same stresses that every mom does. They deal with tantrums (I have seen it), they worry that they won't fit into their pre-baby jeans (I have heard about it, and worse), and they ache for more sleep and more hours in the day. Do yourself a giant favor: Just focus on you and your family and making your home the happiest environment. The rest will fall into place. Pretty soon you will be the one the other moms are looking at and wondering what your secret is.

There is this one mother I am acquainted with who is "perfect." Now, I do not mind this "perfection" at all. In fact, I sort of welcome it because my child benefits from the crafts and activities that she does.

My child came home from her house once and gleefully said, "Did you know you can sew buttons BACK ON YOUR CLOTHES?!?" Like it was the greatest secret ever. Honestly, how else would my child ever learn that. Well, yes, I suppose I could sew, but what use would we have for safety pins?

—Chris Jordan,
blogger, NotesFromTheTrenches.com

I'm not Supermom, I know I'm not perfect—far from it—and actually, I don't try to be. One of the most important lessons I've learned over the past eighteen years is that not only is it impossible to be Supermom, I don't want to be.

I am important, as a woman and an individual, not simply as a mother and wife. I've learned that if a woman gives up one aspect of herself—the woman in her, the mother, or the wife—the other facets suffer. Often women think the opposite: that if they just concentrate on being good mothers (preferably, perfect mothers) then they'll automatically be good women and wives. Nothing could be further from the truth. A woman must be aware of herself and her needs so she can be aware of the needs of her family. Women don't need to feel guilty about taking care of themselves, because it will only help them to do a better job of caring for others. You must take care of yourself first for everyone else's sake, as well as for your own.

You owe it to yourself to focus on finding the way to your own heart. I believe that every woman regardless of how many roles she juggles not only has the power to be in control of her life but has the innate ability to pull it all off with great aplomb and joy.

—Kathryn Sansone,
author of *Woman First, Family Always*
and happily married Hot Mom of TEN!

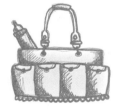

The soul that has no established aim loses itself.
—Michel de Montaigne

Find Your Passion

Our kids can be our greatest inspiration. Now that you have decided to carve some time for you, spend it doing something you feel excited about. Motherhood broadens us and adds strength to our character. It gives us an entirely new perspective on life. Our children open and expand our world in so many ways. And you owe it to your children "to fill you bucket" so you have more to give to them. Go ahead, shine, and make your light bright.

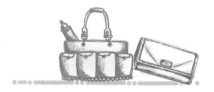

Carl Jung believed our lives need meaning and purpose. He felt that if we don't have meaning and purpose, we acquire bad habits in order to create drama and excitement. Jung called these patterns "low-level spiritual quests."

No Fear

I am thirty-nine years old. I have boys ages eight and twelve. Three years ago I took up freestyle BMX biking—ramps, jumps, peg stalls and more—and I love it! Learning new skills on a bike over time has presented me a learning curve I just can't rush. Through patience, dedication, and new risks, I've found the courage in myself to face some fears and discover new strengths. My boys don't just see my riding as something their mom does; it is part of who their mom is. Their friends are always amazed that a mom could do something like this. (So are their parents.) I just know that age and gender are not an issue for me when pursuing what moves my spirit. So be good to your heart. Live your passion.

—Rochelle L'Italien, BMX mom

Getting a life means getting a life outside your life, a life that really comes from the deepest place inside of you! It's not about adding to your already overflowing schedule. It does take a certain amount of time and commitment to find your creative expression, but it's AMAZING how much more energy you will have when you find something you love to do, for no other reason than that you love to do it. My only advice is if you want to be a Hot Mom for the next fifty years, make sure to take time out to figure out who you are when you take your apron off at night.

—Joy Rose, founder of Mamapalooza

From the second my son Troy was born, everything took a different shade. To realize I had this little being in my arms, that I was responsible for guiding his life, was so awe-inspiring that words can't even describe the feeling. The next year I was completely devoted to mirroring the best of him and imprinting the best of my husband and myself. I chose not to work, except a bit here and there; besides, I was only feeling inspired to be a mother to my son. I really didn't have any type of creativity running through me. That was pretty scary after being a musician my whole life. There were times I thought, Okay, now what? I was a musician for twenty years and now I'm a mother. This is who I am now; will I ever be a musician again? Will I ever want to be? Then I started recharging my creativity in ways I had never experienced. From day one, beautiful melodies would pop into my head and I would just start singing to Troy. Funny songs, too, about what I imagined he was thinking. Cool beats and fun lyrics all in my head, coming from my heart. I started keeping a small recorder next to the rocking chair . . . and there I was, still rocking, just in a different way!

Now, looking back, sixteen months and a new CD later, I realize I was doing what I had always done but in such a profoundly different way I almost didn't trust it. It was so effortless and so inspired. This has been the best writing and recording experience of my entire life, and many have told me it is their favorite record of mine. Being a mom unleashed a newfound artistic freedom unlike any other. Because I was so connected and present with my baby, I organically tapped into another side of my creativity by entering into that innocent world of exploration and wonder.

—Meredith Brooks,
Grammy-nominated recording artist

Doing for others doesn't mean you have done your job. I'm talking about giving our daughters slightly better tools, with a strong united message that we can be even better mothers, wives, daughters, lovers, sisters, and workers when we remember to take time to nourish ourselves in deeply soul-inspired ways. What's inside will shine out. That means spending time experimenting with something that's creatively passionate. Whether it's music, poetry, painting, or dance, do something that makes your body move and your mind engage and your heart leap with the satisfaction that you have participated in bringing forth something utterly lovely from your soul. This is ultimately the core of an inspired life.

> When we agree to bring a child into this world, we facilitate not only the repopulation of our species on some primal level but we also agree to facilitate another human being's fruition of their potential. To do that, we must be actualizing our own potential—not merely through a duty-bound existence matched to our responsibilities but through each of our unique forms of self-expression.
>
> —Joy Rose, founder of Mamapalooza

Get a Life!

Let motherhood inspire you and motivate you to explore your passions. Bring new projects into your life. It is only fitting to talk about beginning new things at the beginning of this book. List all the things you want to start: taking singing lessons, grabbing coffee with the girls, biking, getting a facial once a month, reading for fifteen minutes a day, taking longer showers . . . whatever it is, big or small, start something.

No mom is an island, although some days you may wish you were stranded alone on one. Devote time to seeing other moms and their kids. That will help ease any stress and it will be fun for your kids, too. Motherhood will naturally bring you into a whole new social circle. Today it is easier than ever to find cyber soul sisters and likeminded moms to hang out with. There's a staggering number of blogs and motherhood websites, so you will most certainly find someone who shares your views or whose child shares your toddler's obsession with picking his nose. There was no such thing as Facebook or Parents Connect when my son was born. The Hot Moms Club was started in part to fill that void in networking for moms. Take some time and cruise through a few of our favorite sites and blogs and see which ones feel right to you. Join a playgroup. Socializing is good for you and your kids. The trick is finding parents and kids that you *both* actually enjoy spending time with.

> *As wonderful and nostalgic as it may be to reconnect with old friends, your social possibilities are not limited to the people who knew you when Aqua Net dominated the top half of your head.*
>
> —Joanne Kimes, coauthor of *The Stay-at-Home Martyr*

HERE ARE SOME OF OUR FAVORITE BLOGS AND MOM SITES FOR CONNECTING AND CHATTING.

- ✿ Alphamom.com

- ✿ Babble.com

- ✿ BabyCenter.com

- ✿ BostonMamas.com

- ✿ ClassyMommy.com

- ✿ CoolMom.com

- ❀ Facebook.com (where you can join our Hot Moms Club group)
- ❀ Family.com
- ❀ HotMomsClub.com
- ❀ LilSugar.com
- ❀ ModernMom.com
- ❀ Mom360.com
- ❀ Momfluential.net
- ❀ MomItForward.com
- ❀ MommyTracked.com
- ❀ Momversation.com
- ❀ ParentDish.com
- ❀ ParentsConnect.com
- ❀ PlaygroupsUSA.com
- ❀ RoleMommy.com
- ❀ RookieMoms.com
- ❀ SheKnows.com

The Hot Mom's Handbook

- ✿ SVMoms.com

- ✿ TwitterMoms.com

- ✿ UrbanChild.com

- ✿ YummyMummyClub.ca

There are hundreds of hilarious and incredibly well-written blogs on the Web today. Here are a few of my favorites to add to those listed above. Plus, many of these moms have blogrolls or list other sites they love. It might take a bit of searching, reading, and laughing, but you are sure to stumble upon a blog you connect with and find a new daily favorite.

Baby on Bored, by author Stefanie Wilder-Taylor, is witty and well written but also personal and confessional.

Dooce.com is one of the most popular blogs on the Web. Check it out and see what all the fuss is about.

One of the most controversial mom blogs is **Free-Range Kids,** by Lenore Skenazy, who believes you need to let kids have a life outside the cage and not go nuts with worry. Her tagline is "Commonsense parenting in uncommonly overprotective times."

Jessica Gottlieb's blog is frank, fun, and to the point. If you use Twitter, she was recommended by *Forbes* as a top power mom to follow.

NieNie Dialogues is a blog by Stephanie Aurora Clark Nielson, a mom of four who narrowly survived a small-plane crash in 2008. Despite being left with burns over her entire body, and despite her challenging and extremely painful recovery, Stephanie writes a blog that is uplifting and real. There is no complaining about the difficulties of motherhood. Stephanie is overjoyed to be alive, as she almost lost the chance to watch her children grow up. And although at first she swore she would never post photos of herself on her blog, she has come full circle, sharing family photos and experiences as she did before her accident. She is truly an inspiration, and whether she realizes it or not, she teaches every one of her readers about the beauty of unconditional love for oneself, for life, and for family.

Notes from the Trenches (tagline: "Fighting the war on terror one tantrum at a time") is written by Chris Jordan, who has "more kids than you can count on one hand" and a bigger sense of humor than most people I have met.

Mom-101's tagline is "I don't know what I am doing either." It's written by mommy guru Liz Gumbinner, who is also the cofounder of **Cool Mom Picks**.

Mominatrix, a column on the website **Imperfect Parent.com,** is hilariously written by Kristen Chase, the other founder of Cool Mom Picks. She is also the author of *The Mominatrix's Guide to Sex* and writes the popular blog **Motherhood Uncensored**. I love Kristen's tell-it-like-it-is style—there's no holding back and no topic is off limits.

Motherlode is a blog by *New York Times* contributor, author, and mom extraordinaire Lisa Belkin.

Got MILPs?

Everybody has heard of MILFs (Moms I'd Like to F**k). However, MILFs technically only comprise a small subcategory belonging to a larger, umbrella group of über-annoying moms I like to call MILPs (Moms I'd Like to Punch).

Who are MILPs?

MILPs are a growing group of annoying, offensive moms who are a menace to the general population of weary moms innocently minding their own business, and just trying to survive till the next nap. Their sole mission in life is to make your life harder and to question your own judgment, while advancing their own evil mom agendas. While most MILPs are merely clueless, self-absorbed and insecure, the most hardened MILPs can be judgmental, obnoxious, intrusive and downright dangerous.

Here's a list of the worst offenders:

MILFs

MILFs are the most minor offenders because they're usually too self-involved with maintaining their MILFiness to take notice of you. Being a hardcore MILF is hard work and time-consuming. All the hair appointments, working out, the mani-pedis, the facials, the shopping and dieting doesn't leave much time to spend with their offspring. They're generally too self-absorbed to notice your parenting prowess. Unlike other mom subgroups, they have no interest in trying to convert you to their way of life because, like—OMG!—who needs the competition?

And yes, MILFs are notoriously snippy, since they have chronically low blood sugar from carb deprivation. But they're also easy to spot and easy to avoid. The most annoying thing about them is that they perpetuate the standard of an unrealistic "new normal" for the vast majority of moms with chipped manicures, unwashed hair and a few leftover pounds that won't budge.

Sanctimommies

These sanctimonious, holier-than-thou moms are my archenemies. Yet I'll be the first to admit that I have my own inner sanctimommy moments all the time. This uptight breed of mom can be recognized with their permanently pursed lips, constantly rolling eyes and eyebrows raised in disbelief at your inept parenting. Under the veil of anonymity, these moms get their judgmental fix on the Internet by trolling parenting message boards and persecuting moms who work, circumcise, use pacifiers, don't breastfeed through grade school, don't practice attachment parenting, watch TV, use disposable diapers and don't buy organic. Emboldened by their bully-ing success, some moms graduate to . . .

Drive-By Parents

This mom is known for her hit-and-run style of snarky color commentating. She's that mom in the checkout line at the grocery store who will hiss in disapproval and dismay at the balloon and lollipop you allow the check-out clerk to hand to your toddler by saying, "I hope you know that those are both choking hazards!" and zoom off. These moms are the most insidious because they hastily leave the scene of their crime before the shocked vic-tims can react—or retaliate.

Typhoid Marys

Their kids are always, always sick and they never, ever keep them home from school or play dates. Even if their kids are home with diarrhea and vomiting from the rotavirus, these moms will drop off the homemade muffins lovingly made with their infected hands for the entire class to share at the Christmas party their darlings were forced to miss. Whenever there's an outbreak of any contagion, you can be sure that their kids are patient zero!

Germaphobes

Conversely, these germ vigilantes are the natural enemies of the clueless Typhoid

Marys. They're always on the alert for cooties and will shoot you the stink eye if your child so much as sneezes or farts in their child's general direction. These moms never leave home without Lysol wipes and Purell in their diaper bag and can be seen barking, "Don't touch that!" to their offspring in public restrooms.

Alpha Moms

She's the momager who micromanages every detail of the class holiday party and is quick to smack down any parent who dares to deviate from how she wants things done. She is usually PTA president or room parent at your school and rules her fiefdom with a well-manicured iron fist.

Hovercraft Moms

If she could wind bubble wrap around her child, she would. This quintessentially overprotective mom hovers within striking distance of her offspring and yours (if they dare approach) at all times. She monitors every interaction, poised to intervene if your child so much as crosses their eyes at her precious.

Slactivist Moms

These are the totally inattentive moms at the park who either pretend not to notice and/or simply don't care that their feral, freakishly large-for-their-age hell-spawn are running amok, knocking your toddler down and kicking sand in their face. Yet any attempt on your part to impose order is met with a glacial stare and outright hostility.

Road Warriors

Cocooned in their oversized SUVs, these moms are a menace during drop-off and pick-up times at school. Double-parking, blocking driveways, rear-ending cars with their piss-poor parallel parking skills and hitting pedestrians are all in a day's work. These moms are the most dangerous of MILPs and the traffic cops are never around to slap them with a badly needed citation. They need to put down their lip-gloss wands and cell phones and go back to driving school.

Unfortunately, this is only an abridged compilation of MILPs, since there are oh-so-many more of them out there. What makes me such an expert? Simple. I've been a mom for almost seven years now and I can totally see myself in many of these MILP categories (particularly germaphobe). I've walked a 10-minute mile in their well-heeled shoes and as a rehabilitated MILP, it takes one to know one

—Minsun Park,
Hot Mom of two and blogger,
SheKnows.com

Hello Baby: Good-bye Friends?

As you are creating your new group of mom friends, keep in mind that your relationships with your friends who don't yet have children are about to change as well. If they don't feel this way already it won't be long before your friends (without kids) start to think *you* are preoccupied and boring, fulfilled solely by musings on your offspring, and blind to their imperfections. And guess what: They will be RIGHT. You may feel *they* are thoughtless, self-indulgent, or immature and have no idea what it is like to be up every hour with a newborn. And you will be RIGHT. There is a natural shift in your lifestyle, and although there is a divide in your respective priorities, if you acknowledge and plan, there does not have to be a divide in the friendship, just a tweak in its dynamic. You will have to renegotiate a little bit. Your friends who don't have children may never fully understand until they have kids of their own the trouble you went to just to show up (late), and that you have to leave early (again) to relieve the babysitter. When the relationship becomes unbalanced and one party feels they are putting in more effort than the other, that's when tension arises. Try to involve your friends as much as possible in your new life as a mom, but also make time, even if it is only once a week or twice a month, for coffee with girlfriends and talking about music, movies, politics, shopping, relationships, etc. . . . anything that interested you BC. This will not only please your friends but also help you feel connected and balanced as well.

DADS ARE THE NEW MOMS

Remember, your hubby is going through the same adjustment with his friends. If he is the first of his buddies to have children, that can put a lot of strain on him. It is safe to say his buddies will be less understanding than yours. Women are generally better at making new friends and adjusting to change in their social circles and in life in general. So as a member of the superior gender, try to show compassion for his plight but set up some guidelines to help him carve out time for his friends and still give you the attention you need and deserve. This might be the perfect time to start befriending other cool couples whom you feel like you fit with and who either have kids or have a baby on the way.

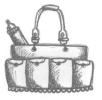

How to Balance Baby with BFFs

Few single experiences can change a woman's life more than having a baby. And as much as our grandmothers, society, our mothers, and other mothers can try and prepare us for the many areas where our lives will morph into something completely different, all due to the sweet little bundle of joy . . . there is little ever mentioned or written about the impact this experience can have on our friendships. See, the girlfriend thing remains steadfast and impervious through everything . . . or so they say. The truth is, however, when a BFF hasn't shared this eternal life-altering experience, there can be tumult, difficulty, tension, and the kind of emotional strain with which we as women can really struggle.

When two women who have formerly had years of friendship without the responsibility of motherhood, the basic adjustment is a big one when one of them has a child. It affects everything from not having the time to talk on the phone, to the entirety of everyday life. My best friend in the whole world had her children later in life; she is presently the mother of two kids under the age of three. She came to my house recently sobbing. When I asked what was the matter, she said, through her tears, "I am so so so sorry, sorry I didn't help you more when your kids were little. I mean

I had no idea how hard it was, and now I feel terrible." There it is: we can't expect a friend who has not had a child to be able to understand the transition. And we shouldn't, so keep your expectations low in that area. . . .

Women who don't have children handle this dynamic differently. Depending on her overall life and contentment level, this can be really hard or somewhat seamless. Remember to factor in the reality of your friend's circumstances and her desires. Much like brides, new mothers can fall into the trap of "sorry but it's all about me." Don't do it—our friends are our safety net, our soul holders. They are some of our greatest sources of strength and support. Keep a keen eye and have faith that you will navigate through this much like everything else you've weathered together, and come out closer, stronger, and with new and different memories together, memories that both of you will someday covet almost more than anything you have thus far experienced. Children are the true telltale of the passage of time, and motherhood can bring an even deeper sense of honor and regard to one of most coveted relationships we as women know . . . friendship.

—Liz Pryor, Hot Mom of three, columnist,
and author of *What Did I Do Wrong?:
When Women Don't Tell Each Other
the Friendship Is Over*

Each day is new. You can wake up tomorrow and start fresh with a new attitude and new way of doing things, take control, and stand firm. The earlier the better. If you don't start a routine or claim time for yourself and do things that nurture your spirit, you will end up like one of those moms on *Supernanny*. So tomorrow, wake up with a smile and a purpose. Find time. Find things you want to do and friends you want to do things with. Decide that you are worth it and that one of the best things you can do for your family is to be at your best.

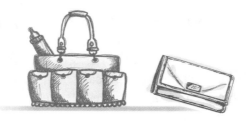

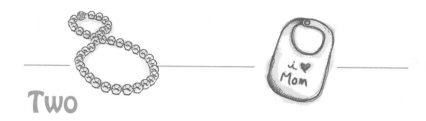

Two

Wake Up Your Sleeping Beauty

*I know this is going to sound corny,
but I first became happy with the way I look
when I became a mother.*

—Angelina Jolie

The very first secret is that it is healthy to want to feel hot and desirable. It is okay to enjoy and honor who you were made to be—a HOT MOM! Before you can become a Hot Mom, you have to admit that you want to be one. We've been conditioned to feel that it's wrong to want to be hot after we become moms, that it somehow works against our abilities as a mother. HA! I am telling you that it is normal to want to maintain elements of your former self, your sexiness your desirability. Keeping this part of you on ENHANCES your abilities as a mother, a lover, and a friend. We have been so brainwashed to believe that moms can't be sexy, that their lives must revolve around their children, that that's what a "good" mom does. For decades we

> Wake up the Hot Mom inside you! *It's all about attitude.*

have accepted the idea that once a woman becomes a mom she shouldn't be sexy anymore. I can't think of anything more ridiculous. Who said we must become frumpy after we have children in order to show our dedication to motherhood? Unfortunately, it's easy to fall into this trap. Society seems to say *You're a mother now* in a way that implies that a good mother has no time to care for herself.

> You're not just the "mother of some child." You're not just "someone's wife/girlfriend." You're not just "some company's female executive." You're that wild child from high school, that cocky rebel from your early twenties. Remember her? She's there, just waiting to come out. You can still nurture and take care of your beautiful babies. You can still be the respectable member of the PTA and the ladies' power lunch club, but do it with the new haircut and nails. Throw on a pair of heels, honey, and low-slung Joe's Jeans—just don't lose your badass. Don't lose your outlaw. Don't lose the fiery, sultry woman inside of you who lives life to its fullest with kids in tow, eyes aflame, and hair blowing in the wind.
>
> —Sheila Kelley, creator of the S Factor

Being a Hot Mom has nothing to do with age, race, size, or situation and EVERYTHING to do with attitude. There is nothing sexier than confidence. A Hot Mom exudes it. I can't say this enough: Confidence is what makes it happen. Self-esteem is one of the greatest gifts you can give your children, and they will learn it best by watching you. Our children mirror us; they watch how we live and how we carry ourselves, and they imitate us in ways you may not even be aware of. So remember, confidence shows in the way you walk, the way you talk, and the way you care for yourself. We are all intrigued by and drawn to confident people. Confidence is power. Confidence will gain you the respect of your children and make your man want you like nothing else. This has to come from within. You can't look to anyone else to give you confidence because they can take it away as quickly as they gave it. It's a process, and every exercise in this book will boost your self-esteem and inner strength.

> If I could wave a magic wand, confidence is the gift I would give every woman in this world. It is the first thing that every woman needs in order to be sexy, especially moms. Confidence is what makes a mom hot. Confidence makes a woman rock. With so many people to care for and so much to juggle, it is a mom's confidence that will see her through when all else fails. You must develop a rock-solid sense of yourself. A woman can't feel good about herself if she is always focusing on what is wrong with her. If all you see is every little dimple on your thigh or extra inch on your waist, it will be difficult to have confidence. So you have got to start by being your own best friend.
>
> —Eve Michaels, image consultant

If you want to be a Hot Mom, decide right now that you are. It's just that simple. It comes down to choice. You have a right to choose what type of woman you want to be after you have children; you just have to truly decide it. Being hot begins in your mind. So wrap your head around the fact that it is okay—more than that, it's healthy—to want to be hot.

I am one HOT MOM!

That's it. That is the most important thing in this book: the decision to be a Hot Mom. What you tell yourself, you believe; what you believe, you become, and this affects how you feel and how you treat yourself, your children, husband, friends etc.

Put this book down and shout, "I AM ONE HOT MOM!!" Go on, do it, and say it with *attitude*. Say it again and again. Say it in your head:

I am one hot mom. I am one hot mom. I am one hot mom. I am one hot mom. . . .

Yell it at the top of your lungs. "I AM ONE HOT MOM!!!!" Sing it. "*I am one Hot Mom, oh yeah yeah yeah.*" Inform all of your friends and family (and maybe even a few strangers) that they are in the presence of a Hot Mom. Say it every day, every hour, for as long as it takes until you truly, sincerely OWN IT. Insist that people introduce you as Billy's Hot Mom, write HOT MOM in lipstick on your mirror, have business cards made up that say JENNIFER, HOT MOM OF _____ (list your kids). If this seems silly, good! Hot Moms are silly. Hot Moms don't take the world or themselves so seriously.

Call it your mantra, call it your affirmation, call it whatever you want, but whatever you do, starting right now, call yourself a Hot Mom. If you really want to be a

Hot Mom you must commit to it. We all say we want things, but it is not until we commit to them in our hearts and our heads that we will achieve them. Hot Moms don't do anything halfway.

I know, I know. Your body isn't the same after having one kid or five kids. Of course not! Your body has performed one of the most awe-inspiring human feats. With supermodels like Gisele in every magazine and billboard flaunting their bikini-clad bodies only months after giving birth, it's tough to maintain a healthy self-image, even before your body has been stretched and reshaped and kicked from the inside. It has taken me a long time, but I've realized that the way you perceive yourself is more important than the way others perceive you. Unfortunately, most women have a false self-image.

Living in Los Angeles, I have met some of the most beautiful women in the world, literally, and guess what? They have asked me if their butt looks too fat in their jeans, complained that their arms are too long, their noses are too big, or their ears stick out. I've heard it all and thought, "Are you kidding me? You are walking perfection! How on earth can you feel this way?"

So, you are probably wondering, What does this have to do with me as a mother? EVERYTHING. The way your children feel about their bodies all comes from you. So if you don't like who you are or the way you look, how can you expect them to like who they are or the way they look?

A Hot Mom is a mother who has confidence and raises her children with values and tons of love. A confident mother is a confident child.
—Carnie Wilson, singer and songwriter

Just the Way You Are

My son has thick hair and two crazy cowlicks, and no matter what gel or mousse I use, by the end of the day his hair goes in a hundred different directions. I find it adorable. I purposely keep his hair long because I love it so much. It's unique to him and always makes me smile. My hair also has a mind of its own; however, I don't always find it so cute when it won't cooperate.

One day my son saw me struggling to flatten a piece of my hair. He came up next to me and started flattening his own hair. He kept getting more and more frustrated when it wouldn't hold into place. I told him I loved his hair just the way it is. Then he turned to me and said, "Mom, I love your hair just the way it is." Wow. His words hit me hard.

Self-confidence is the X factor of life. It has a long-term impact, and little things can make a huge difference. We owe it to our children to fall in love with ourselves, just as we are. Commit to loving what you've been given and loving what you have done with it. It's time to love the shape of your hips, the gap between your teeth, the fact that no one in the whole wide world looks like you and never will. Love your uniqueness, your imperfections. Love being twenty-six, thirty-one, forty-five, or eighty. Love the age that

> *If you pour your energy into what you don't have you'll have nothing. Pour it into what you do have and the world will lay itself at your feet.*
>
> —Joy Rose,
> founder of Mamapalooza

you are and the wisdom you have gained. Know—and I mean really know—how special you are.

Get Naked

That's right, you heard me. Put this book down. Go to the mirror and STRIP. Take off ALL OF YOUR CLOTHES. Look at yourself—really look at yourself—and BE KIND. Our bodies have been criticized, judged, and rejected by us for years. Today and every day moving forward you are going to focus on your assets and discover new qualities. Look at and acknowledge your new curving hips or beautiful breasts, love the definition in your arms, or the color of your eyes, or your beautiful hair, or your cute little toes. The more willing you are to do this, the easier it will become. Go with this mantra: *My body is more beautiful than ever.* Say it again: *My body is more beautiful than ever!* Say it every day. Every time you get into the shower, say it and believe it: *My body is more beautiful than ever.* Your body will respond to this appreciation and grow increasingly more beautiful. You will feel lighter, you will glow, you will truly be astounded by the effects of loving your body.

Remember, if you are not comfortable with your body, how can you expect anyone else to be? Get right to the heart of it, your naked self.

The most perfect thing about us is that we are imperfect.
—Goldie Hawn

Walk around naked tonight in your bedroom, walk around naked tomorrow night, be naked as much as you can until you are truly comfortable in your own skin.

Photographs

As moms we are always behind the lens snapping shots of our adorable offspring, only once in a while jumping in a shot. When was the last time you had a photo shoot for just you? For your high school yearbook? About six years ago a fashion photographer friend of mine suggested we do a shoot for fun, and I reluctantly agreed. At first looking at the photos all I could see were the flaws and the bad angles. But the more I shot, the more comfortable I became. I found you get the best pictures when you let yourself go and leave your self open. It took hundreds of shots (literally), but eventually I was able to relax. As with anything, it takes time to loosen up and adjust your thinking about it. Getting yourself photographed will absolutely build your self-esteem. You should capture your beauty on film regularly. The more pictures you see of yourself, the more you will enjoy seeing pictures of yourself, and the better the pictures will be. It's all conditioning and training. Love your body; capture its beauty on film. Your hubby will love the photos as well. They make a great gift—but more on that in chapter 7 (wink, wink).

Acknowledge Your Fantasticness

I cannot overstate the importance of acknowledging your body and its specialness, your absolute exceptionality. Your primary relationship in life is with yourself; all other relationships reflect this. The more your learn to love and appreciate yourself, the more love and appreciation you will receive. How you feel about yourself determines the quality of your life, your relationships, your healing, and capacity to succeed. As much and as deeply as you love your children, it is equally important to fall madly, unabashedly in love with yourself! If you love every ounce of your being, you will naturally teach your children to love themselves the same way. So value your fantasticness—I am not sure if that is even a word, but it fits and I am using it. You can find fantasticness in EVERYONE.

Take a few minutes and think about what makes you fantastic and put it down on paper. It may be difficult at first; we often feel awkward stating anything positive about ourselves. Tell me what your best asset is. Do you have Michelle Obama arms, a killer smile, bright eyes, a tight butt, an infectious laugh, good boobs? What is your best feature, what are you most proud of?

The more your confidence builds, the easier it will be to write a list of things you love about yourself. Write what you can for now, then each week you must discover an amazing, fabulous new part of yourself and add it to that list. Keep adding to that list until you need a new piece of paper or even a new notebook. This may seem a little silly, but it really works. There is something very liberating about acknowledging your incredible self and being proud enough to write it down.

When I was a student teacher at a junior high school, we did an exercise that was really well received. I had each student write their name on the top of a piece of paper and number down to twenty-three—the number of students in the class. As they passed the papers around they each had to write (anonymously) something positive about the person whose name was on the sheet. Afterward, several of the kids came up to me beaming that they didn't realized other kids noticed certain things about them. Some of the kids kept their lists in their wallets. Start a list for your kids of the top thirteen things you love about them, and then have them write the top thirteen things they love about themselves. You can take it a step further and send it to grandparents and relatives, or do this at a Thanksgiving or holiday party. As I wrote this section I stopped to send an e-mail to my man telling him the top thirteen things I love about him. He was surprised and touched; we always say how much we love each other, but we rarely list the reasons or the specific qualities we love. This is a good place to pause, put this book down, and do the same, for your kids, your parents, your husband, a friend, and even yourself. There is no downside to telling the people you care about how special they are and why.

So make it a habit to write and acknowledge the things you love about yourself. Acknowledge and write down the fantastic things about the people closest to you. The more you focus on the beauty of other people, the more you will start to hone in and focus on your own beauty and strengths. Look for the specialness in your friends, family, and children and be sure to tell them often. Never underestimate the power of a sincere compliment. Pay attention to what you say. Are you dishing out compliments or criticisms? Count how many compliments you give in a day and how many complaints you make about people. Today, really make an effort to notice the uniqueness and wonder in EVERYONE you come in contact with. Focusing on the positive externally will make it easy and natural to focus on the positive internally. So be quick with a compliment, be sincere, and for every compliment you receive, give three. Can you imagine if everyone did that?

Compliments

I read somewhere that compliments are contagious. I hope that's true. As I mention above, it is important to give at least three people a compliment each day. It is not hard to do this. When you are looking for something great in people, you will always find something; maybe the girl at the post office has beautiful eyes, or maybe you love the color of that woman's scarf—and no mother gets tired of hearing how wonderful her child is. Just be sincere; say only what you mean or feel. If you are thinking it, why not say it? It's easy to find special things in the people you interact with. They say we need to hear something positive ten times to believe it's true, but something negative only once. It is also said that one insult can wipe out a hundred compliments. Why is the negative stuff easier to believe? The problem is that many of us (myself included) don't give enough compliments to the people we come in contact with, and especially not enough to the people we care about. We are often quick to criticize and slow to compliment. Let's make a pact and reverse that trend. It's proven that compliments increase a person's self-esteem and cause people to feel happier.

Be especially mindful of your words when speaking to your kids. Their self-esteem is even more fragile than ours.

Before I started the Hot Moms Club, I was a private teacher and tutor for the children of movie stars, professional athletes, and some very wealthy families. I was working with a thirteen-year-old girl who was an accomplished equestrian. We were on location for six weeks for one of her tournaments, and while we were away I noticed she hardly ate anything. She confided to me that she felt fat. I should preface this by saying she was adorable, and maybe a size 4 or 6. I made it my mission to build her confidence, and after a month of constant reassurance I had made progress. She was feeling happier, and when we were out to dinner she would eat confidently. Then, for her brother's birthday, her parents chartered a small plane to fly us home for the night so she could attend the party and still be back the next day for competitions. We walked in to the event and were greeted by her grandmother, whose very first words were, "It looks like you gained some weight!" My mouth almost fell open. In four seconds this woman had undone

My mom never saw the irony in calling me a son of a bitch.

—Jack Nicholson

the positive self-image I had worked for a month to build. I noticed the rest of the night that the girl picked at her food. She ate some veggies and passed on cake. It broke my heart.

Your criticism may not be so obvious, but be cautious and mindful of what you say. Sometimes our words or comments are subtle and uncalculated, but it doesn't mean they don't affect our kids' self-esteem. Once I was supposed to do a photo shoot with my son. The day before, he was at his dad's house, which was near the hairdresser. I asked his dad if he could take him in for a quick trim, just clean up the back and sides so that he would be ready for photos. When I picked him up the morning of the shoot, my son had a buzz cut. Literally, his entire head was shaved, with only the tiniest hairs sticking up. From afar he looked bald. My first reaction was shock. I was really surprised to see him this way because his hair was long and full for years. Admittedly, I was upset, and I couldn't hide my emotion. I had a vision of what I thought the photos should look like, and I said without thinking, "What happened? I really wanted these photos to be great." My son said, "Why won't they look great now?" He started rubbing his head, and I could tell he was suddenly feeling self-conscious. I felt like an A1 jerk; throw me in mom jail and toss away the key. I quickly apologized and explained that I was just surprised. I said they *were* going to be great because now we could really see his cute face. Luckily, I had caught myself, but how many times do we make a quick comment like that?

Why We Feel the Way We Feel

What would your life be like if you always felt confident?

Do you remember an adult or teacher who built your confidence—or crushed it? You never know the power of your words when you speak to young people. The more positive frame of mind you are in and the more confidence you have in yourself, the more positive your interactions will be with your kids.

I remember dropping my son off at school once during testing, and as he was getting out of the car in the morning, I said, "Good luck today! You are so smart, you are going to do great!" His reply was, "Mom, I know, I know—I'm smart, I'm kind, I'm handsome . . ." I hope he always feels that way about himself. As he closed the door, I smiled and yelled, "Don't forget modest!" and he said, "What's 'modest'?"

They say we have roughly sixty thousand internal thoughts a day. We control whether those thoughts are positive or negative.

Thinking is your self-talk, your internal dialogue, which influences your emotions. Your emotional state influences your behavior, which influences the results you see in your career, with your family, and in society. If you can change your thinking from negative to positive, you

People are like stained-glass windows. They sparkle and shine when the sun is out, but when the darkness sets in, their true beauty is revealed only if there is a light from within.

—Elisabeth Kübler-Ross

can change your feelings and your environment in a positive way. And although confidence starts on the inside, with you, it also requires outside help.

Sometimes looking back can help you move forward. Think back to when you were young, to a teacher or an adult who influenced your confidence by either building it up or knocking it down.

I still remember one year in grade school, feeling petrified all summer that I would get a certain teacher who was old, mean, and bitter. Sure enough, the first day of school, she called my name for her class. My mom says I looked ghost white. One day during the first week, I had to go to the bathroom really bad, and I was too nervous to raise my hand and ask. At some point another girl asked to go and the teacher barked, "Fine." It gave me the courage, so timidly, I raised my hand and asked to use the restroom. She rolled her eyes and said in a snarky voice, "Monkey see, monkey do." I was mortified . . . and afraid to raise my hand in class the whole year for anything.

For a Quick Confidence Boost, Make Improvements You Can See

Get a new haircut or color, get your nails done, buy new makeup—it's up to you. Even a new lip gloss will make you feel more confident immediately! I don't know anyone whose self-esteem doesn't increase after they improve how they look. For those of you who think this makes you too self-important, I say get over that fast! I don't know a single person who doesn't leave the salon without that "I can take over the world" attitude. It sounds silly, but it's true. Look at your children and see how they strut after a haircut or wearing a new outfit. The truth is, looking better makes you feel better, and it's that end result that matters. Your outside should reflect your inside. And conversely when you are feeling good on the inside you want to reflect that in your appearance, in how you look, walk, and talk. As you take better care of your spirit, you will naturally want to take better care of your self in all areas. We were not born out of style. We get that way when we stop putting effort into our appearance. Your appearance, makeup, hair and clothes are as important as your smile. When you project an image of confidence, you set yourself up for success (and, in turn, you set your children up for success). Treat yourself with respect and other people will treat you with respect—and you will teach your kids self-respect. The hardest part is the beginning, deciding you are worth the effort of keeping yourself up and deciding to allow time in your day to do it. The truth is, it really doesn't take as much time to maintain ourselves as we think. The hardest part is getting past the ridiculous notion that doing so somehow makes us vain. A healthy attitude starts on the inside, knowing and owning it; the next step is showing it. Others' response to you will only reaffirm your feelings of self-worth.

A positive self-image is a crucial part of our emotional well-being. A negative self-image can lead to a negative attitude. I experienced this firsthand. I fell into the "I'm too busy to" trap. I let myself go out of convenience and I used my son as the excuse. I never had time. The truth is, we always make time for the things we really want and need to do.

Give your appearance the attention it deserves, because you deserve it! Taking a few minutes a day to get yourself together is not impossible if you make it a priority. Get creative. Love having your nails done? Grab the latest color of the season and take ten minutes after the kids have gone to bed and apply it. Or incorporate it into your day. Set a time and paint your nails with your daughters, or set your son up with a paint set of his own.

The more pride you take in your appearance, the more people will respond to you. It is easier to like someone if she likes herself. The truth is, you are already a Hot Mom. You just have to WAKE HER UP!!!

So get up right now throw on some bracelets with your outfit, pull out those fun earrings you haven't worn in a while—who says you need an occasion to wear special things? *YOU are the occasion.* Try a few of your lipsticks, blow out your hair—whatever it is, make an improvement that you and others can see. It's amazing

Priority: (n) Anything that is important to you.

Don't you love it when some incredibly beautiful woman like Linda Evans or Cindy Crawford tells us that the real beauty secret is finding your inner light? Right. But I've done the same things these woman have done to find my inner light, and while it's true I am happier, I still don't look like them.
—Marianne Williamson

what this does for your psyche. Do a little today and do a little more tomorrow. Make this a habit!

These tips may not turn you into a supermodel, but they will help you look your best. Everyone's basic primping routine is different. There are women who would never dream of leaving the house without putting on makeup or using a few different hair appliances. There are others who might easily leave the house wearing two different shoes. The trick is finding the balance and what works and makes you presentable. Being around so many Hollywood pros, I've picked up a few great beauty tricks here and there. I hope these MEs (Mom Essentials) help you look and feel your best.

Let's start with some great news: You don't need to spend a fortune and you don't need fancy Beverly Hills doctors. Many of the best beauty tricks are things you can do at home. One of the most wonderful skin care treatments is available to everyone. It doesn't just make your skin glow but benefits your whole body, and is utterly painless to use. It's called water, and you drink it. Drinking water increases your energy, and it brightens and clears your eyes and complexion. Drinking enough water also relieves bloating and puffiness. Water carries nutrients to every cell in your body, flushes out toxins, and improves circulation and blood flow.

How many times have you heard, "Drink eight glasses of water a day"? I know what you're thinking: You can barely keep track of your car keys, let alone how many glasses of water you drink. But like it or not, hydration is vitally important. Most people are in a state of mild dehydration. Did you know that the human body is about 60 percent water? The brain itself is about 75 percent water and is extremely sensitive to dehydration. Dehydration effects your mood, your energy level, and also your complexion. Many people think that tea, coffee, and soda count toward the daily water needs of the body. Although these drinks contain water, they also contain dehydrating substances such as caffeine, which counteracts their hydrating properties. So when you drink caffeinated coffee, tea, or soda, your body may expel more water than you're taking in.

If you are like me and forget or find it challenging to drink enough water, you will need to make an extra effort. I came up with a few tricks to help make this easier—and tastier. If keeping track of eight glasses seems too overwhelming, buy a liter-size water bottle and drink two a day; that's much simpler to manage. If you get bored with plain water, try a delicious flavored water, like Hint, a brand of naturally flavored water with no sweeteners or preservatives. The peppermint is my favorite. You could also invest in a clear pitcher that can hold two liters or more, fill it with filtered water, and—if you want, for fun (just like at the spa)—drop in thinly sliced lemons, limes, oranges, and cucumbers. Throughout the day, pour yourself water from your pitcher. When the pitcher is empty, you've had the proper amount. Adding frozen fruit like kiwi, peach, orange, apricot, or plum instead of ice cubes will also make any plain glass of water more fun and refreshing. The frozen fruit looks colorful and cools your drink while giving it a bit of flavor.

H₂ Ought Oh

It is very important that you filter your tap water. According to studies, more than 315 pollutants can be found in the tap water we drink. (Visit the Environmental Working Group's website, EWG.org, to see how clean your city's water is and to find information about filtration.) There are various types of filtration systems that fit right on your faucet as well as portable systems like Brita to keep water clean and fresh. Do your research and select the best one for you.

Bottled water is more popular than ever. Just beware and be conscious that the composition of many plastic water bottles includes bisphenol-A (BPA), a potent chemical that mimics estrogen in the body. Studies have found that freezing, heating, or reusing the plastic water bottles can cause the BPA to leach into your water. Refillable stainless steel bottles are a safe alternative.

ECO-MINDED MAMA

No more plastic bottles! The Intak, by Thermos, is a BPA-free refillable water bottle. It has a built-in filter, and the cap is numbered and rotates so you can keep track of how much water you are drinking.

Considering the amount of water you and your family will be downing, purchasing a few reusable thermoses or stainless steel water bottles (for around ten dollars each) is cheaper in the long run then buying plastic-bottled water. If you have a refillable bottle already, put eight rubber bands (if it holds eight ounces; use fewer if it holds more) around it in the morning and take one off each time you refill it. That is a quick and cheap solution that will help you keep track of the number of glasses you drink during the day.

Sleeping Beauty

Experts say you need eight hours of sleep a night. When you are sleeping you are getting more than just rest; your body is repairing and healing itself. And lack of sleep doesn't just cause puffy, red eyes or dark circles. When we are tired we release the stress hormone cortisol. High cortisol causes (among other things) the breakdown of collagen in skin.

> *Anyone who says "sleeps like a baby" clearly doesn't have one.*
> —A new mother

Well, sleep is one of the biggest luxuries we as moms miss. Rest to relax, nap to revive, and sleep to rejuvenate. Resting can even be that five- to fifteen-minute break of literally just putting your feet up while your baby is sleeping or at school. Perhaps you can catch up on your favorite magazines or listen to music, but whatever choice you make, let yourself relax into a comfortable chair and refuse to run for anything, not even the phone.

Naps. I'm a type A personality, and not the type that would even consider sleeping during the day, but whenever I indulge in a fifteen- to thirty-minute snooze, I am shocked at how much more energy I have. So allow yourself the luxury of taking a short, refreshing nap every day. Sometimes this takes some self-convincing, because we're women and no matter how tired we are, we will always think of at least a dozen things we could be doing. Nap when your children do. If you just can't bring yourself to nap, try meditating.

Just keep in mind that napping for longer than thirty minutes or an hour actually puts you into deeper stages of sleep, which can be hard to awaken from and can leave you feeling groggy rather than recharged.

Sleep or Not

While I consider waking up with your baby a parent's rite of passage, there are some measures you can take that will help your child get a good night's sleep and you get your beauty rest. Let your baby or kid sleep in his own crib or room. Set a specific bedtime for him and stick to it. Babies and kids thrive and feel safe with routine.

Create a sleep ritual. When my son was a baby I would sing "You Are My Sunshine" to him every time, without fail, when he went to sleep or I saw he was getting sleepy. It wasn't long before he unconsciously associated this song with closing his eyes. It worked like a charm. To this day (and my son is now ten years old) if I see that he is getting anxious or not feeling well, I sing that song and it instantly relaxes and calms him. Pick a song to sing or play, read a story, or anything else you can do every night to create a sleep ritual and signal that it's bedtime. When your child sleeps, you are able to sleep, and sleep is crucial to helping you feel and look your best.

Quick Tips to Cure Tired Eyes

Cool cucumbers, ice-cold spoons, or frozen tea bags are all remedies. It's the cold that reduces the swelling. Beauty pageant contestants and many makeup artists I know swear that carefully dabbing Preparation H (yes, the hemorrhoid cream) under the eyes removes the bags. It acts as a vasoconstrictor, relieving the swelling. I have never personally tried this, but many women I know say it is magic.

$TUFF TO DROOL OVER

There are many agencies that specialize in night nannies, who work specifically during the night, usually for the first six to ten weeks after your baby is born, so you can sleep. Prices range from $20 to $40 an hour, and the rate varies depending on the number of children. The use of night nannies has risen dramatically in the past five years, especially in big cities and among families with multiple births.

Smile

One of the best beauty tips is to smile. It makes your beauty barometer shoot way up. We are generally attracted to and feel more comfortable with people who are smiling. Let's face it, we would rather look at someone who is smiling and beaming than someone who is frowning. Smiling people appear more confident. And the best part is that smiling affects your emotions. You actually feel better when you smile. So start right now. Smile—see? You look better already!

A tip for having a brighter, more beautiful smile is tooth whitening. White, bright teeth can make you look years younger, and tooth whitening has become affordable for almost everyone. Talk to your dentist about his or her prices and look on your supermarket or drugstore shelves for white strips. Remember, coffee, tea, wine, and fruit juices can stain your teeth.

I don't believe makeup and the right hairstyle alone can make a woman beautiful. The most radiant woman in the room is the one full of life and experience.
—Sharon Stone

BABY ON A BUDGET

Brushing with baking soda is a great way to keep your teeth white and bright.

ECO-MINDED MAMA

Strawberries actually contain an enzyme that whitens your teeth. Mash strawberries in a bowl, then rub them on your teeth with your finger for a minute and rinse and floss. Voilà!

Body Brushing

You already make a habit of brushing your teeth; here is something to add to your morning routine. I have recently started this, and I have to say I love it: dry brushing my body. Every day I take my round body brush ($12 from the Body Shop) and run it over my arms, legs, shoulders, and back. It feels so good, like an internal massage, and it takes less than a minute. My son loves it, too. There are many benefits to brushing your body. It removes the dead skin layers, strengthens your immune system, tightens the skin, stimulates circulation, and (they say) helps remove cellulite. It's inexpensive and invigorating. Our skin is the last organ to receive nutrients from the body and the first to show the signs of deficiency. It only takes a minute—literally—to make sure you are exfoliating and taking care of your skin, and the results can be dramatic.

Celebrities make beauty seem effortless, but I promise you, a lot of work goes into making them look natural. I am sharing with you some inside tips and secrets from some of the most well-respected makeup artists and stylists in the business. Many of these regimes and products I use personally or have personal experience with. My goal is to help you feel as confident and radiant as possible.

Let's Face It

Like me, most moms are so exhausted at night it's a wonder they ever manage to wash up before bed. But exfoliation is one task worth staying up for, and it only takes a minute. When you have a healthy, glowing face, everyone takes notice. As we age, our skin doesn't shed dead skin cells as fast as it used to, so it can look dull and flaky instead of vibrant and smooth. Exfoliation gives your skin a boost and increases circulation as well as collagen production.

There are many affordable scrubs you can use daily. At the Hot Moms Club, we love:

❀ Aveeno Skin Brightening Daily Scrub. It uses soy extracts and smooth microbeads.

❀ Olay Regenerist Micro-Derm Cleansing Cloths. Wet the cloth and work around your face, using the bumpy side first, then finish with the smooth side.

❀ Neutrogena Deep Clean Gentle Scrub.
Microbeads exfoliate and beta hydroxy
cleans.

❀ Fenix Green Tea Exfoliating Scrub. It works
on age spots and has botanical extracts to
lighten and tone skin all over.

❀ Sircuit Skin Sir Active. Small jojoba beads
exfoliate while the zeolites (silicates from
volcanoes) remove impurities.

BABY ON A BUDGET

Brown sugar works great as an exfoliant. Keep some in
a sealed container or Ziploc bag in your bathroom, and
the next time you bath, grab a handful, lather, and gently
scrub your face, arms, and body. You can mix the sugar
with olive oil as well—it helps revitalize skin. Use olive
oil on your elbows, too, to keep them from cracking and
drying out.

Freshen Up

Being in the public eye, celebrity moms always need
their skin to look baby fresh. Part of their regime is to get
monthly exfoliating facials and trips to the dermatologist for professional microdermabrasion treatments. It

works, but how many moms have the time or the budget to do this? NuBrilliance sells a microdermabrasion machine for home use. Although it is more expensive than most creams, it's less expensive than professional treatments and is just as effective. It costs about the same as one treatment in a dermatologist's office.

No matter what way you choose to exfoliate, make sure you do it! It is the cornerstone of fresh, vibrant looking skin.

Keeping your skin hydrated is also an important part of an anti-aging regimen. Beauty mists made from mineral water are wonderfully refreshing to apply, especially in the spring and summer months. They also revive your makeup during the day. Evian Brumisateur Mineral Water Spray comes in travel sizes, which are perfect for riding on airplanes, when your skin is more likely to get dried out. I also love the Vitamin E Face Mist from the Body Shop. My son loves it when I spritz him during long flights. It helps refresh our skin and our mood.

$TUFF TO DROOL OVER

Colorescience Setting Mist (Colorescience.com, $35) is a facial spray that comes in a variety of formulas. It helps set makeup, hydrates, and refreshes your face. Molecular Mist by Sircuit Skin (SircuitSkin.com, $36 for 2 ounces) is ultra hydrating.

Create your own mist with ingredients you already have at home. There are many different types of mists. You can experiment with your favorite herbs. Take two cups of water (preferably mineral water), add a green tea bag or two, and a small spoonful of honey. Boil, then remove from heat and let steep. Strain and pour into a spray bottle and refrigerate overnight. (This keeps for one to two weeks.)

Eye Eye Eye

What a difference perfectly groomed eyebrows make. They open your eyes and add symmetry to your face. Well-groomed eyebrows can make your whole appearance more sophisticated and put together.

Go to a professional at your beauty salon for an initial eyebrow shaping and consultation. Then maintain that shape by tweezing.

The ideal shape for your eyebrow is not a C or an arc, a thin line or a comma. Eyebrows should form a straight angle up and back toward the natural arch then taper down slightly at the outside corners.

The best time to pluck is right after your shower, when your pores are open.

Even when features are asymmetrical—as they most often are—well-shaped brows will bring a kind of harmony to the face.
—Anastasia Soare, the "Eyebrow Guru" (Anastasia.net), a favorite of countless celebrities, including Oprah

That makes tweezing easier and less painful. Remember to pluck unwanted hairs in the direction of the hair growth; pulling the opposite way can cause red bumps. Remove plucked hairs from tweezers frequently for the best grip, and don't forget to sanitize the ends of your tweezers with a cotton swab dipped in antiseptic or rubbing alcohol before each use. Fill in any gaps or uneven areas in the eyebrow with a brush using an eye shadow one shade lighter than your hair color. Be careful not to use too much; otherwise, the end result will look unnatural.

Another quick tip that takes only a second and instantly opens and brightens your eyes: Curl your eyelashes. Eyelash curlers cost around $4, and curled lashes really make your eyes pop. Hold and count ten seconds. To really hold the lashes in place, warm the curler first with a hairdryer. (Test the curler on your hand to make sure it is just warm, not hot.)

$TUFF TO DROOL OVER

One of the best-kept secrets and latest beauty obsessions in Hollywood is eyelash extensions. They add length, thickness, and fullness to natural eyelashes. The lash extensions are applied one by one to the existing lash, not to the skin, and each eye takes between thirty and eighty extensions. Each extension lasts as long as the natural growth cycle, which is approximately two months, sometimes even three. The procedure takes and average of one to two hours, and prices range from $150 to $500 per set.

For a night out or special occasion, try Ardell Fashion Lashes. They've been around for years and are a fun staple for any makeup collection. At only $3 a packet, they usually last one or two days, and you can apply at home.

Kiss and Makeup

I advise every mom to update her makeup bag. Take your most stylish friend or relative and visit a department store like Macy's that has various makeup counters and make an appointment for a consultation. The makeup consultant will help customize a look based on your needs and help you choose the right products and colors for your skin type. You are not obligated to purchase any of the products; you may want to get a few there and get the rest at the drugstore. It's important to know what works for you. Once you have your staples, you can update them with a fresh new lip gloss or eye shadow each season.

> *I don't understand how a woman can leave the house without fixing herself up a little— if only out of politeness.*
> —Coco Chanel

Once you figure out how to put your makeup on, remember to never fall asleep without taking it off! This is a must. No matter how tired you are, wash your face thoroughly. Your skin needs to breathe and regenerate. Leaving makeup on during the night will clog your pores and cause breakouts.

Baby wipes (especially if they are hypoallergenic and fragrance free) make great makeup removers!

Lip Service

Your lips need to be kissable, both for your partner and for your adorable kids.

Lips gloss is a great way to keep a natural look while adding shine and fullness to your lips. Shimmering gloss both reflects light and enhances the fullness of your lips. To create the illusion of a fuller smile, trace the outer edges of your lips with a neutral liner, fill in with a peachy or rosy color (avoid colors that are too dark), then trace only the V at the top of your lip and the middle of your bottom lip with a liner that is a shade or two lighter than your lipstick or gloss. Remember, dark colors call attention to your lips, so wear soft pinks or colors that enhance your natural color for a beautiful everyday look.

The skin on the lips is very thin and is prone to sunburn. Look for balms that have an SPF of at least 15. A favorite is Kiss My Face lip balms, which have sunscreen and are made from organic beeswax and aloe vera. They have yummy flavors to choose from and only cost about $3. They're perfect for you and for the kids. I always wear ChapStick, too. I keep it in my car, my purse, the bathroom, my desk drawer. (Clear lip balm also makes great moisturizer for your cuticles.)

To prevent your lipstick or lip gloss from melting in the summer, store it in the refrigerator. If you are planning a day at the beach, you can pop your lipstick in the freezer and bring with you. It will be refreshing and keep its shape.

Hair to Dye For

Joy Bergin is a cofounder of the Hot Moms Club and beauty expert who was a stylist for *Entertainment To-night*, *Access Hollywood*, and *The Insider* and has done hair and makeup for top celeb moms including Tori Spelling, Jennie Garth, Jane Seymour, Mary Louise Parker, Denise Richards, and many others. Joy gives her secrets to fabulous hair on a mom's schedule without the Hollywood price tag: "Invest in a great haircut from a nice salon. Get recommendations from friends, neighbors, or coworkers who have great hair. I know it's not always practical or affordable to go to the salon all the time, but starting with the right cut and style for your face is important. You may be able to get away with trims and upkeep at more reasonable place every two months. If you are like me and have dark hair with gray coming in, you know it is not always practical or budget friendly to hit the salon every three to four weeks to cover some gray."

Applying Hair Color Like a Pro

If you choose to do your color at home, take off all of your jewelry (you never think you will make a mess, but trust me, you will), change into old clothes (I have designated hair-coloring clothes I use every time), and switch the bathmat for an old towel. (You can use the same towel to wrap your hair after rinsing out the color.) Pick out a color you like, and don't be afraid to mix a color from a different box to get the desired shade. Most box color comes with 30- or 40-volume peroxide developer, which strips your natural hair of its color and can make it brassy. Instead, buy a 20-volume L'Oréal Oreor Creme developer, available at any beauty supply store. It costs about $3 for a large bottle, which will last you several color treatments. Dump out the developer that comes with the kit and refill the bottle with the same amount of the 20-volume developer. Then mix the developer and color as directed. You can also add shampoo to the mixture; this dilutes the intensity of the developer and gives you more product to work with if you have longer hair.

Make sure everything is mixed well before you apply. Divide your hair into four sections. Separating the front and back and sides with big clips, begin with the first section and work along the root line. Leave the color on the roots for thirty to thirty-five minutes. In the last fifteen to twenty minutes, work the color through the rest of your hair. Wash, rinse, and blow dry!

BABY ON A BUDGET

Mascara is a quick fix for covering a few gray hairs. Use brown or black depending on your hair tone to help hold you over until your next appointment.

Find a beauty college or teaching salon. Students pass their tests by learning on real people. If you sit for them you can usually get your cut and color for free. They usually work under the supervision of a professional, so it's worth inquiring and researching.

Taking Care of Your Locks

Once a week mix a little bit of baking soda with your shampoo to get a really deep clean. The baking soda will help remove built-up product residue. Add a handful of baking soda to a sinkful of warm water and soak your brushes and combs to wash out any residue from hair products.

It's best if you wash your hair every other day or every two or three days. This will make your color last longer and won't dry out your scalp. If your scalp starts to get too oily, apply baby powder to the roots of your hair, bangs and all. It will be absorbed.

If you hair is naturally oily, use conditioner only on the bottom half of your hair, as if you are taking out a ponytail. That way you can detangle your hair without making it too heavy or oily.

To give hair an extra-shiny and silky texture, apply a mixture white vinegar and water, let it sit for five to ten minutes, then rinse. Gorgeous!

Mayonnaise is another great budget-friendly way to restore hair's moisture and add shine. Just apply the mayo, wait ten to twenty minutes, then wash and dry as you normally do. Voilà! Why does this work, you ask? Because eggs, oil, and vinegar—the three main ingredients in mayonnaise—moisturize and add sheen.

Hair spray is great for holding hair in place, but most sprays use many chemicals. A natural way to make hairspray is simply combining sugar and water. Boil water, remove from heat, then add two tablespoons of sugar and stir. When it cools, pour it into a spray bottle and spray with a very fine mist setting. If you just want a light hold, add more water; if you want that full '80s Jersey prom look, add more sugar. Don't worry, it isn't stiff and it isn't sticky. You can add some lavender oil if you'd like a little scent. It should hold all day, and the sugar water will also add shine to your hair. (The mixture will last for about a week, then you will need to make a new batch.)

Ponytails with a Twist

Ponytails are convenient; they're easy and keep the hair out of your face. But taking an extra second can transform your ponytail from a quick afterthought to a style statement. Brush your hair and pull it back in a ponytail with an elastic band as your normally would, then pull out a strand of hair and wrap it around the elastic until you can't see it anymore, and use a bobby pin to tuck the strand underneath. This is popular with the celebrities. It looks classy and polished, and it couldn't be simpler to do. A side ponytail is a variation that's suitable for longer hair, and it adds an element of style. Brush hair to one side of your shoulder, twist, and wrap it in an elastic band. Braids are also very popular, but if you can't braid your own hair, brush your hair back into a ponytail and wrap with an elastic, then an inch from your first elastic wrap another one, and an inch below that wrap another, and then another, all the way to the bottom of your hair. For another fun look that's easier than braids, you can twist pieces in the front and pin them back with bobby pins.

Unwanted Hair

I'm Italian, so my hair is dark and it grows fast. Shaving my legs and underarms was a tedious daily chore. Two years ago I got laser hair removal treatments and I couldn't be happier. It's pricey; treatments range from $80 to $250 each, and you need to go for several treatments before all of the hair is gone. Many medical spas and dermatologists offer packages and deals, so if this is something you are interested in, look for specials and coupons. It's painful, so most treatment plans include a numbing cream, which I recommend. It's applied forty-five minutes prior to your treatment and will make the procedure a lot more tolerable. After a few treatments you get used to it and it doesn't hurt as much.

Rather stick with shaving? Experiment with razors until you find the right one for you. To get a smooth shave devoid of nicks, be sure to change your razors or cartridges on a regular basis. Make sure to exfoliate before you shave to remove the dead skin that could clog up your razor. Keihl's Simply Mahvelous Legs Shave Cream ($16 at Keihls.com) is great. It has allantoin and chamomile to sooth the skin while moisturizing. Keihl's Close Shavers ($18) is a favorite of several men I know, and it works well on a woman's skin, too.

Baby oil and hair conditioner also work well as shave creams. Conditioner softens the unwanted hair and moisturizes your skin, so no body lotion is necessary afterward.

Throw a Penny in the Fountain of Youth

Our kids keep us young and make us old at the same time. You are never too young to start an anti-aging regime. I am all about prevention. Like my mother and I am sure your mother has told you, wear sunscreen every day. Choose a moisturizer with SPF so you don't even have to think about it.

Experts say nothing gives away your age like your hands. Their skin is thin and delicate, and we often forget to take care of it. Your hands are the part of your body you use the most, so be sure to moisturize them three to four times a day. I usually keep hand moisturizer within reach. Once a week, use your facial exfoliant and your good face cream on your hands before you go to sleep at night.

Head, Shoulders, Knees, and TOES

I have to admit, I absolutely love getting my nails done. It always makes me feel so clean and put together. A good pedicure can last me four to six weeks. I bring my own polish to the salon so that if it chips afterward I can touch it up at home, allowing more time in between visits. OPI has a huge selection of colors. (Find retailers at OPI.com.) I always use clear polish on my fingernails because it is easier to maintain.

Remember, you use your hands more anything else, and they're very visible. There are many very affordable do-it-yourself manicure and pedicure kits and products on the market that cost usually about the same as one visit to the salon. However you choose to do it, keeping your nails groomed is an important element of your appearance. So trim your hangnails and make an effort keep your polish neat.

$TUFF TO DROOL OVER

Chanel and Yves Saint Laurent both offer unique, limited-edition nail polish colors each season, available at fine department stores for $20 to $25 a bottle.

Give Me a Hand

When my son was younger, he didn't like having his nails trimmed, so I tried to make nail clipping a ritual. I picked the same day each week so he was prepared. I filled warm bowls of sudsy water for our feet and smaller bowls for our hands, just like at the spa. We each put our feet in our bowls, and while I clipped one hand, I had his other hand soaking in the warm, lovely smelling water. Afterward, I slathered his legs and arms with moisturizing creams. This ritual turned it into a fun experience and he came to really enjoy it. Sometime later, he was at his dad's house, and his dad went to cut his nails. My son said, "Wait, what about the bubbly water?" I had some explaining to do!

Makes Scents

Smelling a scent you like triggers positive emotions. Find a body wash, spray, and lotion that is pleasing to you but not overwhelming. There are many yummy flavors to choose from. Vanilla is said to be attractive to men, and lavender is said to have a calming effect on children. Suave has a great Lavender Vanilla body wash in their Naturals collection which sells for only about $3.50.

BABY ON A BUDGET

If your favorite lotion is pricey, mix it with a generic unscented brand to make it last longer.

$TUFF TO DROOL OVER

The Kai product line (KaiFragrance.com) is a celebrity favorite. Among its devotees are Jennifer Garner, Reese Witherspoon, Sharon Stone, and Julia Roberts, to name a few. Its light, soothing scent is one of the most sought-after fragrances today. Kai's body wash and body lotion retail for $33 each, and their body butter sells for $60.

The Mommy Monster

Mud masks are a great way to revitalize your skin. While you may not want to treat your husband to this sight in the evening, a great way to get your cleansing done and amuse the kids is to become the Mommy Monster. When my son was small, I used a green mud mask, and I would chase him around the house when I wore it. He thought I was dressing up for him like the Incredible Hulk, and it was really fun. Ask your dermatologist what mask is best for your skin type.

BABY ON A BUDGET

And you thought mashed bananas were just for baby food. Try a banana anti-wrinkle treatment. Mash up extra bananas, put them on your face as a mask after cleansing, and leave on for fifteen to twenty minutes. Bananas are full of vital nutrients and the fruit acids help slough off dead skin and energize the complexion. You can also add honey or oatmeal.

Just Do It

If you don't have a beauty routine, get one. If you think you don't have time, you're wrong. Looking good and feeling good are critical to being a Hot Mom. You're worth it, and your family is worth it. You are not the best mom until you commit to being the best possible YOU.

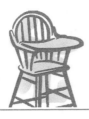

Three

The F* Word—FRUMPY
(Or, Who Says High Chairs and High Heels Don't Mix?)

As to matters of dress, I would recommend one never to be the first in the fashion nor the last out of it.

—John Wesley

Ditch the Sweats!

It's so easy to fall into the comfort rut. It's what I refer to as your "sweats." Sweats represent choosing convenience but sacrificing yourself in the process. It's time to DITCH the SWEATS. I mean that as figuratively as I do literally. A Hot Mom takes charge of her looks and her life. The two work in tandem.

Self-respect: (n)
1. *The proper sense of one's own dignity and integrity.*
2. *Being worthy of esteem or respect.*
3. *Faith and pride in oneself.*

Your outside should reflect your inside. And as you take better care of your spirit, you will naturally want to take better care of yourself in all areas. Let go of how a mom "should" dress and dress the way that best reflects you. What you wear is as important as your makeup, hair, and smile. Projecting confidence and competence sets you up for success in all areas.

As you get more comfortable with your body and inner essence, you will want to express this in the way you dress. Let's face it, it's hard to feel hot when you are covered in head to toe sweats. Now, I'm not suggesting you prance around all day in heels, gown, and a feather boa, but let your outside reflect your inside and wear clothes that show off who you are. Take pride in your appearance. Is your wardrobe telling the world that you don't care? Is that the message you want to send out?

> *My mother taught me to walk proud and tall as if the world was mine.*
> —Sophia Loren

Perpetual Pajamas

Like it or not, every day, 24-7, our appearance gives all sorts of information. The clothes we wear, the way we style our hair, and how we put ourselves together communicate more than words can say. So wear clothes that make you look and feel attractive. This doesn't mean that you have to be uncomfortable, but wearing your husband's oversized T-shirts or ragged old sweats will not do anything for your self-esteem. So forge your own path with your style, but avoid a style rut. While it's good to have a signature look that people identify as yours, do try and change it up now and then.

> *Create your own visual style . . .*
> *Let it be unique for yourself and*
> *yet identifiable for others.*
> —Orson Welles

Confessions of an Ugg Lover

I like comfortable things. We all do. There is nothing wrong with comfy casual clothes. They help you celebrate everyday moments. But even your basics should be treated with as much thought and attention as the rest of your wardrobe. Think "lazy chic." Your everyday tops and tees should be in new condition, not faded, and make sure you have fun new colors and styles.

HERE ARE SOME OF MY FAVORITE SOURCES FOR BASIC TOPS AND TEES.

❀ AlternativeApparel.com

❀ AmericanApparel.com

❀ MichaelStars.com

❀ NationLTD.com

❀ Splendid.com

❀ Tee-Zone.com (for these and all of my
  favorite T-shirt designers on one site)

❀ Velvet-Tees.com

*NOTHING MOTIVATES ME BETTER TO
WORK OUT OR GET MOVING LIKE A
NEW GYM OUTFIT. HERE ARE MY FAVORITE
PLACES TO FIND CUTE YET FUNCTIONAL WORK-
OUT CLOTHES.*

❀ Athleta.com

❀ Athletica.net

❀ BePresent.com has some of my favorite
  form-fitting workout gear. They incorporate
  the yoga philosophy of the seven chakras
  into the design.

❀ Beyond Yoga, IAmBeyond.com

❀ Danskin.com

❀ DSW.com has name-brand sneakers at dis-
  counted prices.

❀ Gaiam.com

- Lucy.com

- Lululemon.com

- Prana.com

- Reebok.com. I am obsessed with Reebok EasyTone shoes. They really do tone your butt as you walk!

- ShaktiActivewear.com has really unique tops.

- TitleNine.com is named after the law that prohibits gender discrimination in school athletics. The website allows you to shop by activity: yoga, running, tennis, etc.

Post-Baby Fashion Crimes

We've all committed them. Acknowledge that it is time to start fresh.

Out with the Old, In with the YOU

The first place to start is to assess your current wardrobe. Know what you have, what you love, what you need to toss, and what you need to purchase to help you look and feel complete. Go straight to your closet and take out everything you haven't worn in a year. It's time to clean out! That's right, do it, take an afternoon and really comb through the stuff you have accumulated over the months or years or, heaven forbid, decades. Don't be afraid. It's actually quite liberating and can be funny when you realize all that you are holding on to. Get rid of the blazer with the big shoulder pads or those "mom jeans" that have a nine-inch zipper and button under your rib cage. We all know they aren't coming back into style.

It's okay to keep a few things with sentimental value, but don't be scared of letting go. Getting rid of the old makes room for the new. Be brave!

When I organize I bring three bags and fill them accordingly. One is for random things that aren't clothing or shoes. Put those items where they belong in your home and keep them out of your closet. Fill the second bag with shoes or clothes that are torn or soiled or beyond repair. This bag goes right in the trash. The third bag is for clothes that you haven't worn in at least a year. You can work on three sub piles as well: Love it, Hate it, and Maybe. Some items may be too nice to toss—maybe it was something you got on sale but was never quite your style; maybe it just doesn't fit anymore. These items are perfect to bring to your "clean out your closet" party. (More on that in a bit.)

No More Wire Hangers

Switch to wooden ones. Everything looks and lays neater and nicer with wooden hangers. Recycle all wire and mismatched plastic. This is an easy way to bring calm to your closet, plus, it's better for your clothes.

Joy Mangano Huggable Hangers (available at HSN .com) are contoured to fit the shape of your clothes so they won't stretch them out of shape. They are made with non-slip velvet coating to keep clothes from sliding off. My favorite part is that they come in a variety of colors so you can color code your closet.

To keep track of the clothes you are wearing. I have a friend who turns the garment's hanger around every time she wears it. At the end of a year, she gets rid of everything that hasn't been turned. A year is a great benchmark. If you don't feel compelled to pull a garment out as you go through the four seasons, chances are you won't in the future.

Labeling your clothes will help you discover what you have and where it is when you need it. There are many fun ways to label boxes or closet bins. If you are labeling things in plastic containers, use clear computer-printable labels with a romantic font to add a touch of elegance and charm. If you are using cardboard boxes, brush on chalkboard paint so you can write the label in chalk, which makes it easy to erase and relabel as needed. You could also use Mabel's Labels (Mabel.ca), a popular source for customized labels. Label-making machines are another fun option. You can make your labeling project an activity to involve the kids in.

ECO-MINDED MAMA

A great way to store out-of-season clothes is in antique or vintage suitcases. These look decorative stacked under the bed, in your closet, or around your bedroom. If you don't have any of your own, search garage sales and flea markets.

$TUFF TO DROOL OVER

If cleaning your closet is too daunting a task to tackle alone, hire a professional organizer. California Closets (CaliClosets.com), despite its name, has locations all over the country.

Shop in Your Own Closet

Invite your most stylish and fashion-savvy friend or relative over to help you go through your wardrobe. She can help you rework and reassess the clothes you do have and reinforce your decisions about the ones you should give away. Find a great tailor and that long dress could quickly become a more practical shorter dress or a top to put on over jeans. Be creative, or have someone creative help you find new ways to wear items you already have. Keep only the items that flatter you and make you feel good. Hold on to things of sentimental value, but otherwise don't be scared to LET GO. Getting rid of the old makes room for the new. Remember, you're a Hot Mom and it's time to create yourself. Style is all about knowing who you are, being proud of that person, and expressing her in any way you feel comfortable. And remember the golden rule of fashion: The way your clothes fit is more important than the tag that hangs inside them. Fit is everything. Know what works best on your body.

BABY ON A BUDGET

What Not to Wear, on TLC, is a great show. Stacy London and Clinton Kelly clean out the closets of wardrobe-challenged women and help them shop for clothes that fit well and look fabulous. Watch and pick up lots of great wardrobe tips and ideas—or apply to be on the show and have your closet overhauled.

ECO-MINDED MAMA

Go green—and get some green! Sell your clothes to a secondhand store. CrossRoads Trading Co. Recycled Fashion (CrossRoadsTrading.com) has locations in many major metros. You can sell your clothes or trade them in for some fresh "new" pieces.

Hire an expert: Wardrobe consultants will audit your closet, help you shop, and give you an entire image overhaul. Sessions vary in price, but most services start at around $125 an hour. Try NewYorkImageConsultant. com in New York City and StyledByLaurie.com in L.A.

Barbra Horowitz, a personal stylist (BarbraHorowitz .com), is known for her unique talent for turning ordinary clothes and T-shirts into masterpieces and works of fashion art. Her specialty is taking what you already have and bringing it new life. Don't live in L.A.? You are in luck: Barbra does Web and Skype consultations as well.

Fashion Meltdowns Are Us

Each season I generally have a few go-to outfits for events and nights out, things that work for all occasions. I have so many different groups of friends and associates I can usually get away with wearing the same few outfits. Not too long ago I was out at business dinner wearing a cute dress I loved and a necklace I had just purchased. You know the feeling when you are wearing something you feel great in? That was me. I was excited because it was also the perfect outfit for an event at my son's school the following night. Well, wouldn't you know it, a group of moms from the school came in, of all the restaurants in Los Angeles, and were seated not far from our table. They saw me and we all hugged and said hello. As I sat back down my face could barely conceal how bummed I was. When I explained my reaction to the other guests at the table, the men couldn't understand what was the big deal, but the woman got it. They know what a pain it is to find just the right shoes, dress, jewelry, etc. Since these moms saw me in the outfit, I clearly couldn't wear it again the following night. I went to the school event wearing something different, and funny enough, as I arrived one of the moms I had seen the night before came right up to me to say hello, and before I could even say anything, she murmured defensively, "I know I am wearing the same outfit as last night, but it's my only nice spring top." The thing is, I didn't even remember what she had had on the night before. But how ironic, I thought, we women are all the same! Even celebrity moms worry about what they are going to wear to various events. A friend of mine who is a mom and an established actress will use a stylist for big events and award shows but will wear only her own clothes for TV interviews and charity events. She often stresses beforehand about what she's going to wear, and rightfully so, with cameras everywhere just waiting to catch her in a fashion faux pas. I remember once suggesting a beautiful dress from her closet, and she said, "That dress is so bright and bold, if I wear it on that show I might as well toss it in the trash. If I get photographed in it again, the tabloid magazines will all make comments." Now, those are high-level problems to have. But my point is that everyone feels insecure at times about looking just right for events big and small. The best thing you can do is know your size, your style, and what garments look best on you and have a few go-to outfits that you feel fabulous in for each season.

Throw a "Clean Out Your Closet" Party

Hot Moms are resourceful and love to recycle. If the thought of paring down your possessions overwhelms you, host a "clean out your closet" party. I throw one every season. I give all of my friends two weeks to prune their clothes and drawers. Then we all get together at my place with our bags of clothes and exchange. It's a blast! We have a little wine, some chocolate, and a lot of laughs. It's always amusing to watch other people part with things they haven't worn in years and tell stories about how and where they wore it. I love watching my friends try to sell each other on something they don't want anymore. The best part: Everyone ends up going home with something "new" to add to her wardrobe, and whatever is left gets donated to a women's shelter. This turns a tedious task into something to look forward to.

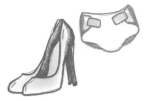

Shop It Out

Treat yourself to some new things. It's okay, you deserve it, so quit feeling guilty. Just because you are a mom doesn't mean you can't keep up your sense of style or create a new one. Hot Moms try new colors and cuts. And don't ever let the thoughts "I'm a mom" or "I'm too old for that" stop you from buying something you really like. Your wardrobe should reflect your attitude, your confidence, and your sense of fun and adventure. Wardrobe shopping is a great opportunity to express who you are. Remember, you can baby-proof any outfit and find a way to let who you are shine through any clothing choice.

> *In matters of style, swim with the current; in matters of principle, stand like a rock.*
> —Thomas Jefferson

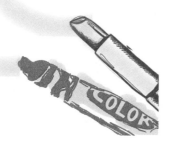

Do You Have a Closet Full of Nothing to Wear . . . ?

As the mother of two budding fashion plates, I take my role as a Hot Mom very seriously. In addition to wanting to look good for me and my husband, I want to set an example for my girls that fun and fashion don't have to end once you have started a family. Looking good is important for girls of all ages, but somehow it seemed much easier to pull it all together without someone pulling on your best sweater and turning your favorite tank top into the perfect gown to wear while trying out their new paint set.

I hear it all the time from my friends who are moms: there's no time to shop anymore, and if there is, you somehow find yourself gravitating more towards grabbing that comfy 6X instead of your sexy size 6. And then of course, some of those former 6s just don't fit the way they used to. Isn't it easier to stick to a uniform of ratty jeans and a comfy sweater if your kid is just going to squirt their juice box on it anyway?

My answer is a resounding NO! C'mon, you didn't start eating food from a jar just because your baby did, did you? So why would you settle for looking drab and boring when there are so many better options?

—Carilyn Vaile, stylist and designer

A CliffsNotes Closet

If you are one of those moms who feel really over-whelmed by the idea of putting together a presentable look, I have a solution. For those five minutes in the morning when you are tempted to default to the sweats and tees, I suggest that the Hot Mom have a quick go-to area or "CliffsNotes" version of her closet. This is where you can keep the outfits and items you can turn to in an emergency to achieve Hot Mom status. These pieces should be tried and true, easily accessible, and ready at a moment's notice. Comfortable dresses are perfect to keep in this area since they take no time to put on—allowing you more time to play with your accessories and shoes!

> Style is an expression of individualism mixed with charisma.
> —John Fairchild

Juicy Couture reinvented the tracksuit, making it sexy and stylish. Flattering on most figures, it is comfortable but still keeps you looking and feeling put together. This is the perfect go-to outfit to keep in your CliffsNotes closet. Victoria's Secret also has adorable hoodie-and-pants sets at affordable prices.

The Hot Mom's Style Arsenal

You don't have to invest tons of time and money—just set aside a little of each to develop your secret weapon: the Hot Mom's arsenal of wardrobe essentials. Essentials are trend-proof. They never go out of style and can be worn with anything. These pieces are flexible, too, meaning you can easily change the entire look by adding a couple of accessories.

Bad-Girl Panties

When building a house you always need to start with a solid foundation; the same is true with your wardrobe. Begin with a fabulous foundation. Underneath every Hot Mom's outfit you will find some sexy underwear. Don't worry, we're not saying you need to give up all your comfy cotton bras and undies. But every mom occasionally faces a situation where she wants to feel like more than a mom, and the best place to begin is

Shapewear: (n)
A foundation garment
such as shaping
underwear designed
to temporarily alter
the wearer's body shape
to achieve a more
fashionable figure.

with what you can't see. It is remarkable how sexy wearing a pair of red lace thongs can make you feel.

Did you know approximately 85 percent of all woman are wearing the wrong bra size? The right bra will make you feel more comfortable and will help you look better in your clothes. Intimacy, a company founded by Susan Nethero (who is also known as the Bra Whisperer), has helped clients including Oprah and the Queen of England. Through its stores and website, MyIntimacy.com, Intimacy offers free bra makeovers and carries a selection of bras from size A through K.

Thanks to Hot Milk Lingerie (HotMilkLingerie
.com) and Condessa (CondessaInc.com) you can still
have sexy and über-stylish lingerie while you are nursing.

If you are thinking of adding Professional Spanx
Wearer to your résumé, you are not alone. Most women
and many celebrity moms I know wear some form of
shapewear.

Proper shapewear is one of the best wardrobe investments you can make. It will help boost your confidence when you are wearing your favorite outfits. Spanx
(Spanx.com) now has body shaping and slimming
swimsuits and apparel. The Spanx Bod-A-Bing apparel
collection has slimming liners and offers easy black classic pieces that would be key to any wardrobe.

Sassybax's Pretty collection (Sassybax.com) has
shapewear so beautiful, you won't believe it's shapewear.

Glamourmom.com offers nursing bras built in to
a tummy-controlled tank top that you can wear with
jeans or yoga pants.

Reebok (Reebok.com) has a new line of workout
shapewear.

ShaToBu.com offers a body slimmer that shapes,
tones, and burns calories when you wear it. Developed
by a doctor, it incorporates resistance bands into shapewear and is literally a workout that you wear.

Tummy wraps and shapewear are wonderful for taming
and shrinking a post-baby belly. Some of my favorites are
Belly Bandit (BellyBandit.com), Wink (WinkBellyBands
.com), and Tauts (available at BabooshBaby.com).

You can find all the top shapewear brands and a wide
selection of bras and panties at BareNecessities.com.

Mom Jeans Should Be Illegal

No matter where she lives or what she does, every Hot Mom needs a pair of good jeans. In recent years, denim has become dressier, and you simply must have at least one pair that you can slip on (or these days, squeeze in to holding your breath as you use a pair of pliers to pull up the zipper) to feel young, cool, and sexy. You also need jeans to wear around the house, but these too should fit in a flattering way. There's nothing wrong with boyfriend jeans, as long as you don't actually look like him when you wear them. You're a woman and you should be proud of it, so add a funky belt to show off that waist—or to hide a slight tummy bulge—and you're good to go.

If you find a pair of jeans that you love and that fit well, buy an extra pair or two. White jeans for the summer and black jeans in the winter can make any top look dressier and still feel comfortable enough to wear to the park or school pickup. MyTrueFit.com has a variety of top designer denim brands and will help guide you to the right style for your body type. They also have a section which highlights the jeans your favorite celebrities are sporting.

A Classic Black Dress

Think classic, simple, elegant, and versatile—a dress that with the right change of accessories or a colorful cardigan can be worn for almost any occasion, including a wedding, last-minute dinner invitation, cocktail party, business meeting, or date. Having that standby any season/any occasion dress gives you a ready answer to "What I am going to wear to this?" EDressMe.com has a huge selection of dresses for every occasion. You are sure to find one or two or ten that you like.

Wrap It Up

A wrap dress is one of the most flattering styles for most women. Whether a solid or a print, it is the perfect casual outfit. Diane von Furstenberg (DVF.com) is the queen of this style. Invest in a good quality wrap as your go-to casual dress, perfect for baby showers and birthday parties. Wear with sandals or pumps, or in winter toss on tights, knee-high boots, and a cardigan.

The Perfect Cardigan Sweater

A colorful solid or print cardigan sweater is a must. Layered properly it can carry you through all seasons. Wear it over dresses or with jeans or leggings. Add a few sparkly accessories and you are ready for any occasion. J. Crew and Vince.com have my favorite selections.

Fun Flats

Find a pair of flats that will work with both jeans and dresses. They should be both fun and comfortable. Tory Burch (ToryBurch.com) made her mark in the fashion world with her signature Reva ballerina flats. Zappos.com and Overstock.com have many similar classic styles at affordable prices.

Just Fabulous (JustFab.com) is a shoe and bag of the

month club. You take a personality quiz to determine your style, and each month you're sent a list of dozens of shoes and bags you might like to buy. It's like having personal shoppers and stylists on a budget.

> *The only rule is, don't be boring and dress cute wherever you go. Life is too short to blend in.*
> —Paris Hilton

Accessories: The Icing on the Cake

It is the little accents to your wardrobe that confer Hot Mom status: newsboy hats, individualized fashion jewelry, gorgeous scarves tied with a special flair. These little additions go beyond the basics and are essential to a Hot Mom's wardrobe because they can make "basic" look anything but.

It is through accessories that your style becomes unique. Maybe you love using baroque pins to fasten your blazer—whatever seems fun to you will brighten up any outfit. Acquiring a variety of pieces may take some time, but that is the fun part. It's a great excuse to play dress-up, just like we did when we were kids.

Sunglasses are the new mascara, and they're probably one of the fastest ways to add confidence. Big Jackie O glasses are a chic fashion statement and perfect for covering bags under the eyes after your five-week-old keeps you up all night. I encourage moms to go to an upscale department store and talk to the sales girl in the sunglasses department. Work with a pro and she will help you discover which style, size, and tint is best for your face. Then if the sunglasses there are too pricey, you can find same style from a more affordable brand.

The addition of a scarf, either tied loosely around your neck or looped around your waist, can instantly make you feel as if you are strolling the streets of Paris rather than shopping the diaper aisle at Walmart. Scarfology.com has affordable fashion scarves in a variety of fabrics and styles. Visit ShopStyle.com, plug in "scarves," and hundreds of pages of options from all different sites and designers will be displayed; you can sort by color or fabric as well to narrow down your choices.

A cocktail ring is a great way to feel a little in vogue and add glitz and movie-star glam to a simple outfit. Cocktail rings are in style and most stores have lots of pretty options. You can easily find some bling in any price range. Stella & Dot jewelry (StellaDot.com) is a favorite of celebrities such as Debra Messing, Rachael Ray, and Penélope Cruz. They have eye-catching cocktail rings starting at $30.

Take note from my four-year-old daughter. I love watching her play dress-up. She puts her outfits together with such care and she has no inhibitions. I guarantee you will never hear a young girl turn down a feather boa with the excuse, "That's not really me." She knows it can be her at any moment, and something else will be her the next. She inspires me so much, but I also know that the way I dress influences her enormously. Our children learn from our examples. When your daughter sees you not taking the time to bring out your best self, what does that tell her about motherhood? We must set the example of how to be Haute Moms so it becomes innate in our daughters. They deserve it and we are worth it, so don't skimp on the accessories.

—Carilyn Vaile, stylist and designer

"Dress and Tell" Secrets from Celebrity Stylists

Fashion Fixes

A celebrity secret to preventing wardrobe malfunctions is Hollywood Fashion Tape (Hollywood FashionTape.com). Hollywood's product line solves a multitude of problems, from slipping straps to gaping blouse fronts.

No Shows, for concealing nipples, are my absolutely favorite. You can wearing them with your sheerest blouse. (Available at UnderwomanWorld.com.)

SenseLingerie.com has many fashion solutions, from strap clips to bust-enhancing bras and inserts to nipple covers and shapewear.

Lately I've been thinking about how illogical my shopping habits have been. When I buy cheap, unflattering things, I don't actually save money in the long haul. I've been confusing frugality with some twisted, frumpy sense of virtue. I realize now that the most value-conscious choice is to buy things that are well made, that will last . . . and that I love.

Cost per Wear

How many times have we bought something we really didn't love just because it was on sale or seemed like a great deal? Here is a great trick to help you decide what items are worth spending a little more money on: Estimate their cost per wear. Here's an example. I once bought a pair of jeans for $49 on sale. The fit was just okay, but the price was more than 50 percent off, so I got them and proudly treated myself to a latte for finding such a bargain. The only problem was, I wore them once. I just didn't love the way they fit, so in the end I would also take them off and put on my favorites, which cost $195. Although they were a splurge, the fit is perfect and I love the wash. I have had them for two years and wear them constantly. I have easily worn them more than 100 times, so the cost per wear is roughly $1.95. The cost per wear for my "bargain" jeans? A whopping $49. In the long run spending a little more for quality clothes that are timeless and that you absolutely love will serve you better than the so-called bargain that ends up sitting in your closet until it's donated. So estimate how much use you will be getting out of each item and calculate your cost per wear. If you live in a cold climate and you absolutely love a $200 wool coat, get it; you will wear it all season long and for years to come. My winter coat is a classic and I have had it for more than seven years, so my cost per wear has to be pennies by now.

Savvy Shopping Tips and Tricks

Catalog shopping is a great way to get ideas on how to put outfits together even if you don't consider buying anything and even if you can't fit into anything today. Think of it as sort of a creative brainstorming session. Have fun with this. Tear out the outfits you really like and then look for sales on similar items in your price range. Get to know the salespeople at your favorite stores and boutiques; they might tell you when sales are coming up or call or e-mail you when items in your style or pieces you have been looking for arrive. If you can afford to shop there, stores like Nordstrom and Barneys even have personal shoppers. If there's a store you shop at all the time, you may want to consider getting their store credit card. I personally don't use credit cards (frankly, I don't trust myself), but if you pay them off right away and have self control, you can score really great discounts, special promotions, and sales. Save your receipts, too; if you buy something at full price and it goes on sale soon after, many stores will give you the difference, either as a refund or in store credit.

Shopping at the end of the season is the absolute best way to score deals—especially on season-specific items like winter coats and swimsuits. Last year I bought a classic black cashmere turtleneck at 85 percent off. It's timeless. I had to wait to wear it, but I will have it forever.

Color

Color is the first thing people notice in an outfit. It is said that certain colors interact differently with different skin tones. Wearing the right colors for your skin tone can help you appear vibrant, while wearing colors that are not complimentary can make you look pale or washed out. Instinctively we are drawn to colors that look best on us and the colors we feel most confident and comfortable wearing. It is also true the color of our clothes can make us look thinner or larger. Dark colors like black and dark gray are slimming and make us appear taller. Wearing the same color or hue from head to toe also helps us appear svelte. When you don't break up the color, the eye travels up and down the body quickly, creating the appearance of length. You can also use color to help with proportions. We look slimmest when our bodies are in proportion, so wear darker colors on your larger half and lighter colors on your smaller half.

Color is also said to effect mood and attitude, so I say wear the colors you love. Wear what feels good to you and you will then radiate and shine.

WHAT NOT TO WEAR . . . TO HOME DEPOT

✿ If you are petite, go for smaller jewelry and patterns. If you are of a larger build, you can rock chunky jewels.

✿ Make sure that either your dress or bling is the focus, not both. The more ruffles and patterns the dress has, the more simple the jewelry and other accessories should be.

✿ Keep in mind that wearing bright or big, flowery patterns on the biggest areas of your body will only draw attention to them.

✿ Avoid pairing capris and flats. They give the appearance of short, thick legs and a boxy figure.

✿ If you can't hide your chest, flaunt it! Avoid turtlenecks or high necklines. They give a shelflike appearance to your bust, which my friend calls the uniboob. Wear deep V-necks or scoop necks, which elongate your neck. If you are not comfortable showing cleavage, you can always wear a top underneath. Choose necklaces that lie around your collarbone or just above your chest.

✿ Focus on the bottoms first—your pants, skirts, jeans, etc.—when you're shopping. Once you find pieces that you're happy with and fit well, choose three tops to go with each.

A great book on how to choose flattering outfits for your shape is *How to Never Look Fat Again*, by Charla Krupp.

Fits and Fitting Rooms

We all have those experiences of shopping with our kids that involve their screaming and hiding behind fixtures, being desperate to find a big-boy potty in the most inconvenient places, wanting snacks, and of course begging for that $2 ride on the mall merry-go-round. The last time I brought my son shopping with me, he opened the door to the changing room and darted out. I was half dressed and had to hop after him.

> *Today I threatened my children with another marathon session at IKEA if they didn't behave. They begged— "We promise we will be good—don't make us go back to IKEA."*
> —Andrea Jarrell, founder of Hot Mama Ink fashions

The Web:
A Virtual Mall at Your Fingertips

Thankfully online shopping has exploded in the past few years, making it easier than ever to find the designers you love, that certain dress in your size, and deals, deals, deals! You can conveniently shop early in the morning before the kids wake up, while they're at school, during their nap, or late at night. Designer discount and sample sites are amazing for stocking up on basics or getting classic or trendy pieces within your budget. You have to be savvy and visit early, but the discounts make it well worth the effort.

HERE ARE SOME GREAT SITES TO BROWSE, SHOP, AND SPEND YOUR HARD-EARNED MONEY ON.

✿ BoutiqueToYou.com allows you to conveniently shop your favorite celebrity styles.

✿ Chictopia.com has a "people like me" section so you can shop by body type, style, and location.

✿ CoolMomPicks.com is a blog that features items for moms, babies, and kids of all ages.

✿ Couturious.com lets you dress a virtual mannequin before you buy so you can see how an outfit will look put together.

- ❀ **CoutureCandy.com** has all the major designers and a celebrity trend blog so you can track the latest styles and where to get them.

- ❀ **HollywoodHotMoms.com** features celebrity mom styles and where to get them.

- ❀ **Kaboodle.com** lets shoppers post reviews about the best products on the Web.

- ❀ **MomFinds.com** is the sister site to She Finds.com and boasts clothes and brands for baby.

- ❀ **MommiesWithStyle.com** is a blog with the hottest products and styles for moms and kids from maternity to teen years.

- ❀ **Polyvore.com** lets you clip and paste clothes from all over the Web to create complete outfits. You can build your own or browse the ones posted. Contributors and readers alike are quick to help with fashion tips and directions where to find things.

- ❀ **ShopStyle.com** is perfect if you are looking for a specific item of clothing. For example, if you type "black pants," hundreds of brands and designers will come up. You can be general or specific. "Lime green shorts" might garner a few to a dozen hits.

This is the place to go if you are looking for that one item to complete an outfit and don't have time to scour the Web. They do it for you!

❀ **Splendora.com** not only has great fashion finds and trends, but Splendora TV has quick, helpful videos on topics such as the many ways to tie a scarf, fashion violations, etc.

❀ **StyleBakery.com** is a shopping and style site for the "real world." They also have StyleBakeryMom.com for bargains on kids' and maternity duds.

❀ **TheFind.com** allows you to type in any item you are looking for to find all the sites and stores that carry it. It works for coupons as well. It's also available as an application for your iPhone.

❀ **Weardrobe.com** shows current street styles using photographs of people on the street. You can also upload photos of yourself and ask for style advice or comments from the experts and readers.

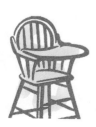

Sign Up for Daily Deals and Visit Discount Sites

These sites boast daily sales that allow everyone access to top designers without the designer price tag, with deals up to 85 percent off retail. (Some require that you register as a member, but membership is usually free.) Warning: You have to act fast. I watch the sites for designers I like and wait for those sales. With prices so low, it can become competitive—and addictive!

- BillionDollarBabes.com
- Gilt.com
- GleeMaster.com
- HauteLook.com
- Ideeli.com
- MamaBargains.com
- Ruelala.com
- Swirl.com
- Zulily.com

*NEWSLETTERS ARE A GREAT WAY
TO STAY FRESH AND CURRENT
ON TRENDS AND PRODUCTS.
HERE ARE A FEW OF MY FAVORITES.*

❀ DailyCandyKids.com

❀ Mamaista.com

❀ Momologie.com

$TUFF TO DROOL OVER

❀ ChickDowntown.com

❀ Net-a-Porter.com

❀ Piperlime.com

❀ RevolveClothing.com

❀ Shopbop.com

BABY ON A BUDGET

❀ BagBorrowOrSteal.com (lets you rent designer bags and jewelry and purchase used
items at deep discounts)

❀ Bluefly.com

❀ H&M (HM.com for store locations)

❀ JCrew.com

❀ NextDirect.com

❀ OldNavy.com

❀ RentTheRunway.com (in partnership with
Us magazine, Rent the Runway allows you
to "Dress Like a Celeb" and borrow dresses
seen on the red carpet)

❀ TheLimited.com

❀ Topshop.com

❀ VictoriasSecret.com

❀ Zara.com

THESE SITES ARE GREAT FOR MOMS WITH A LITTLE FUNKY OR VINTAGE EDGE.

❀ ModCloth.com has a great selection of rare
vintages dresses, jewelry, and clothing.

❀ ShopNastyGal.com has affordable funky
pieces as well as a vintage section.

❀ UrbanOutfitters.com is good for moms with
a hippie chic vibe, and prices are generally
very affordable.

❀ Banana Republic's Heritage collection is
   90 percent sustainable. They use recycled
   packaging and bamboo fabrics.

❀ Beklina.com is an eco boutique specializing
   in sustainable clothes, bags, and accessories.

❀ BTCElements.com has pretty dresses and
   other eco-conscious clothing as well as accessories, such as belts made from bike tires.

❀ EcoStiletto.com is the ultimate resource for
   everything in green trends. Shop, read, and
   win prizes.

❀ GreenWithGlamour.com proves you can go
   green and stay stylish.

❀ Nimli.com has the most beautiful and unique
   selection of eco jewelry from high-end to
   affordable options.

❀ PureDKNY.com features clothing made
   from fabrics like organic cotton, linen, and
   recycled nylon.

❀ TheGreenLoop.com features dozens of eco
   designers, including A Lot to Say (ALotToSay
   .com), which makes T-shirts, totes, baby blankets, and other products from recycled water
   bottles.

❀ Tobi.com has a section on its site called Eco-Tobi devoted to eco designers. The site also has personal stylists on call to help you as you shop the site.

Make Mine a Mei Tai

Wearing your baby has become the ultimate style statement. Baby carriers have become so chic, and they're great for keeping your baby close but your hands free. Admittedly I never did this when my son was a baby. It always seemed he was too big and I was not coordinated enough to work out the carriers. A lot has changed in ten years, and I am very impressed with some of the products on the market today. They are not only functional and easy to use, but they look great as well.

Baby-wearing is not only convenient for parents; according to a study in 1986 by a team of pediatricians in Montreal, it's good for babies. The study found that babies who are carried in baby slings cry at least 40 percent less than those who are unslinged. And the anecdotal evidence is overwhelming: In cultures where baby slings are the norm, crying is measured in minutes, not hours, and colicky or fussy babies are incredibly rare.

Gestation is in fact an eighteen-month experience; it includes the first nine months spent in the new outside world. Because a baby sling carry so closely mimics the feeling of being in the womb, babies immediately begin connecting past and present dots. Sling babies have been shown to be more organized, more aware, and even more in tune with adult interaction than other infants.

If you choose to wear your baby, why not make a fashion statement doing it?* Here are some of my favorite sources, which offer a variety of styles and prices:

- ❀ BabyHawk.com, $80–$140

- ❀ ChicPapoose.com, $68

- ❀ DivasNBabes.com, $89. Their colorful reversible ring slings allow you to both carry your baby and nurse discreetly in public.

- ❀ Lillebaby, $99. Go to Lillebaby.com to find retailers.

- ❀ PolkaDotPapoose.com, $64

- ❀ SerenaAndLily.com, $129. They have several hippie-chic slings that look great and are machine washable.

One of the carrier brands most requested by celebrity moms is Ergo Baby (ErgoBabyCarrier.com), which has been seen on Julia Roberts and Ellen Pompeo, to name a few. These carriers can be worn on the back, front, or side, and they come in a variety of colors, with convenient pockets and zippers and a sun shade for the baby's head. They have a tradition line and an organic line as

---

* Always consult with a professional about the proper and safe way to carry your baby.

well and range in price from $105 to $148. Their ergonomic design make them comfortable on your back. They also offer a doll-size version so siblings can mirror their parents and carry their dolls and stuffed animals.

Moby Wrap (MobyWrap.com) offers a design with UV protection using the Rayosan process, whereby an invisible dye prevents harmful UVA and UVB from going through the fabric to the baby's delicate skin. Moby Wraps are soft and well made, and their website has instructions and demonstrations on all of the different ways to wear your baby.

Kokopax carriers (Kokopax.com, $99.99–$179.99) have a cotton canvas seat but an anodized aluminum frame that you wear like a backpack.

Beco (BecoBabyCarriers.com, $85–$149) makes several kinds of carriers, including a vest style carrier for both men and women, and a mini version ($29) for little girls to use for dolls.

Mei Tai Baby (MeiTaiBaby.com) lets you choose your own colors and designs, with a big variety of patterns and options, starting at $84. They also offer interchangeable panels with your choice of three fabrics so you can change the look based on your mood or outfit.

Accessories for Your Carriers

Papa's 1Z (PapaProducts.com, $25) is a protective cover for your carrier that slips on like a onesie. It's easy to clean and keeps your carrier clean from drool or spit-up.

Baby, It's Cold Outside

- ❀ The BabyBjörn Comfort Carrier allows you to face the baby forward or backward. The waist belt and padded straps distribute the baby's weight evenly onto your hips and shoulders. At $199, it's a little pricier than the other Björn models, but it is the most comfortable on your back in my opinion and lives up to its name. (Go to BabyBjorn.com to find retailers.)

- ❀ The Peekaru (TogetherBe.com, $79) is a fleece vest that zips over the baby carrier cover for cold weather.

- ❀ The Popover (PopoverBaby.com, $90) keeps your baby toasty in his carrier, stroller, or car seat.

BABY ON A BUDGET

My Little Roo (MyLittleRoo.com, $29.99–$39.99) is a stylish slipcover for your carrier, with adorable prints and designs to choose from. It's an affordable way to make that old or hand-me-down carrier look hip and trendy!

Diaper bags have come a long way since I was pregnant. The choice of designs back then consisted of Winnie the Pooh or plaid. Today the functionality is outstanding, and there are endless options to fit any style. Like your pre-baby purse, your diaper bag will be your biggest accessory, literally attached to your hip for the next year of your life. So do yourself a favor: Invest in one you really love—or add it to your baby shower registry!

HERE'S A LIST OF MY FAVORITES AS WELL AS SOME CELEBRITY MOM FAVORITES IN EVERY PRICE RANGE.

❁ Dante Beatrix bags (BeatrixNY.com, $36–$220) are the ultimate stroller accessory. They have special clips that fasten to the stroller and extend to carry across your body. Marcia Cross has the green peace-sign diaper bag.

❁ Hammitt's Suzy diaper bag ($595) is the ultimate splurge. It's the one chosen by celebrity moms like Angelina Jolie. Go to Hammitt.com to find retailers.

❁ Ju-Ju-Be's Be Prepared bag is perfect for mothers expecting twins. It has color-coded tabs to remind you which pocket is for which child, crumb drains, and more. This bag gives you everything but the kitchen sink. Celeb fans include Britney Spears,

Samantha Harris, and Ali Landry, to name a few (Ju-Ju-Be.com, $150–$200).

❀ Mia Bossi bags are so stylish, you'll want to use yours long after your little one is out of diapers. The Hot Mama bag is a favorite of many celebs including Katie Holmes (MiaBossi.com, $200–$1,210).

❀ Nest diaper bags (NestDiaperBags.com, $150–$340) are a favorite of Heidi Klum and Tori Spelling.

❀ OiOi offers a huge selection of fun styles to fit any taste, from the sporty to the girly-girl (OiOiBabyBags.com, $100–$130). Cate Blanchett called her OiOi bag a godsend.

❀ Petunia Pickle Bottom is a staple among Hollywood moms, including Sheryl Crow, and Jaime Pressly. Petunia is known for her classic feminine styles. Their Cross Town Clutch has a fold-out changing pad and room for a diaper and wipes (Shop.Petunia.com, $175–$350).

❀ Skip Hop as a brand has mastered functionality and style, and their diaper bags are no exception. Their collection (SkipHop.com, $29–$90) is affordable and head turning. Rebecca Romijn uses the Studio Tote bag in chocolate.

❀ Timi & Leslie's Charlie bag in black is the
one Jessica Alba uses. Prices range from $60
to $170. Go to TimiAndLeslie.com to find
retailers.

Diaper Clutch

Goober Baby has gift sets of coordinating changing
mats, changing purses, and holders for all of baby's
supplies in adorable designs. They fit nicely into any
bag or can be used on their own.

Design Your Own Bag

If you would like to create or design your own custom
diaper bag, visit B's Purses at BsPurses.com. You can
choose the lining, fabric, hardware, and handle. Browse
dozens of styles and colors to suit any taste.

BABY ON A BUDGET
JJ Cole offers the best bags for the buck. Their Carry-All
Tote is by far the coolest diaper bag on the market under
$20. Also, their Tactic Changing Purse is in a sense a

diaper clutch. Actress Amanda Peet was seen using this diaper bag (JJColeCollections.com, $19–$69).

The Kemby Sidekick (Kemby.com, $165) is a diaper bag and baby carrier all in one. Use the diaper bag on its own or quickly transform it into a convenient baby carrier. The Kemby Sidekick has several won innovation awards and is the ultimate two for one.

ECO-MINDED MAMA

Fleurville diaper bags (Fleurville.com, $69–$150) come with a unique polyurethane exterior that resists cracking, abrasions, temperature changes, and spills. They offer a wide variety of styles and are a completely green company, using eco-friendly materials as well as business practices. Sarah Jessica Parker and hubby Matthew Broderick both have one.

$TUFF TO DROOL OVER

In 2009, designer Rebecca Minkoff added a diaper bag to her line. The first model was a signature leather bag called Knocked Up, in several trendy colors. Kourtney Kardashian uses a Rebecca Minkoff bag to tote Mason's diapers (RebeccaMinkoff.com, $395–$650).

Hush A Bye Baby's 3-in-1 diaper bags (HushABye BabyProducts.com, $695) are cozy as well as functional, with soft, plush cotton chenille.

Gucci has a line of diaper bags starting at $690 (Gucci.com). Halle Berry has one in brown.

Louis Vuitton is the ultimate in luxury, and their Mini Lin collection of diaper bags (starting at $1,950) is used by Victoria Beckham, among other celebrities.

DADS ARE THE NEW MOMS

Just as there are for moms, there are plenty of diaper bags out there to match every dad's personality. Here are our favorite diaper bag sources for your dude.

- ❁ DadGear.com has cool bags that you can customize with your guy's favorite college sports team. They also have cool fleece jackets with compartments to fit diapers, wipes, and a bottle, which are ideal for outdoor enthusiasts or dads who like cool things. Dad Gear offers something for every type of dad. Their unique variety is perfect for dads with an alternative style as well. Prices range from $80 to $110.

- ❁ DiaperDude.com also has a great selection of diaper bags in masculine colors and patterns such as camouflage and skulls. Prices range from $60 to $145. Brad Pitt has been seen sporting their Black Dragon diaper bag.

- ❁ GooberBaby.com has a Gents line with a preppy, thick-corduroy diaper clutch ($28) for guys who might not want to carry a bag.

- Stork Tools, by Dr. Moz, has a big and sturdy bag—think briefcase for the rugged—for around $50. Go to DrMoz.com to find retailers.

- The Logic bag, by JJ Cole ($34.95), is where fanny pack meets superhero belt, but it slings over the shoulder. It's durable, and the ultimate in practical. Go to JJColeUSA.com to find retailers.

ECO-MINDED MAN

Diaper Dude has an eco-friendly messenger bag called Green Dude (DiaperDude.com, $98) that has the same functionality and style you can expect from the brand, but it's made from recycled PET (plastic water bottles).

Fleurville's Re-Run bag (Fleurville.com, $80) is seriously stylish with superior organization, and it's environmentally friendly to boot. Two thumbs up.

Dad's Baby Case, by Passchal (Passchal.com, $349), is made from black eco-friendly leather and recycled tractor inner tubes. It looks stunning, can easily double as a briefcase, and each one is unique. Blair Underwood has their black messenger bag.

Petunia Pickle Bottom's Rubicon Rucksack messenger tote for him (Shop.Petunia.com, $271), in black or brown leather, is both gorgeous and functional, the ultimate city bag or "man bag."

Storksak, a celebrity favorite of Julia Roberts, Gwyneth Paltrow, and Kate Winslet, to name a few, offers a unisex bag that's made from pebbled leather (Storksak.com, $210). It's masculine, stylish, and designed to fit not only bottles and other baby gear but also a laptop.

Fashion Dos—or Doo-Doos?

There are some interesting and outrageous products on the market today, and at the Hot Moms Club, we have seen it all. For fun, here are a few that you might find amusing. I'll let you decide whether they are a fashion do or doo-doo.

Designer Diapers?

You may have to wiggle to fit into your old jeans, but now your baby can wiggle around in a new pair of denim diapers all day long. Made by Huggies, these are for the baby who wants to look stylish while he's pooping his pants!

Pampers has also launched a designer diaper line,

Pampers by Cynthia Rowley, which features stripes, ruffles, and several unique prints.

Heelarious are soft shoes for baby that are designed to look like high heels (Heelarious.com, $30).

Now your baby can get wiggy with it by wearing a baby toupee. They offer the Bob (baby dreadlocks), the Donald, and the Lil Kim (long pink hair) (BabyToupee.com, $21.99).

Billy-Bob Pacifiers are pacifiers with big buck teeth, vampire fangs, and other designs on the front (BillyBobProducts.com, $5).

ChasingFireflies.com has the cutest selection of unique Halloween costumes for little babies and toddlers ($29–$58).

MyBabyClothesBoutique.com has over-the-top but adorable looks, from big flower hats for girls to baby fedoras and driver caps for boys.

As seen on Suri Cruise: Move over Rachel Zoe. I could probably write a whole book on this little fashionista, and in fact there is already a blog dedicated to Suri's style: Suri Cruise Fashion (SuriCruiseFashion.blogspot.com). One of my favorite looks that Suri rocks is from NoKo. They have Japanese-inspired dresses and little kimonos (NoKoBaby.com).

HERE ARE SOME OTHER ADORABLE BABY SHOPPING SITES AND BLOGS WITH GOOD ADVICE.

❀ Converse.com (Converse now lets you design your own sneakers)

❀ CoolMomPicks.com

- ✿ HollywoodHotMoms.com

- ✿ LesCulottesCourtes.com (for trendy, fashion-forward kids)

- ✿ MasalaBabyNYC.com

- ✿ MightyJunior.com

- ✿ MommiesWithStyle.com

- ✿ SavvyMommy.com

- ✿ ShopKitson.com

- ✿ UpscaleBaby.com

- ✿ VeryMeri.com (where kids can design their own T-shirts)

Hot Wheels for Mom?

I know, I know: Things have changed since you've had babies. Once you were a speed demon, but you are now in jeopardy of being stopped for driving too far under the speed limit. A joy ride now means just going somewhere *without* the kids.

But trading in your sporty coupe or sedan for a minivan doesn't have to be traumatic. Comedian and author Stefanie Wilder Taylor wrote that when she went to purchase her minivan, she felt like a cat on his way to be neutered. But don't fight it; roll with it and rock it out.

Your car may just be your biggest accessory, and as a busy carpooling mom it may feel like your new office, so treat it well. It doesn't matter whether it is old or brand spanking new, take good care of it, don't let the kids trash it, keep it clean. It's good car-ma (sorry, couldn't resist). Just as you de-cluttered your closet, take pride in your car's appearance. It is another representation of who you are. Wash it twice a month. My son loves to go through the drive-through carwash. You could let some neighborhood kids wash it while it's parked in right in your driveway. And as your kids get older, washing the car will be a fun task they will look forward to helping with.

HERE ARE SOME SOURCES FOR CAR SEAT ACCESSORIES TO MAKE YOUR LITTLE ONE LOOK STYLISH RIDING AROUND TOWN.

✿ BabyCarSeats.com

✿ HipNCozy.com

✿ PinkTaffyDesigns.com

✿ RitzyBaby.com

✿ SassyCovers.com

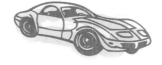

Four

Fewer Pampers, More Pampering—<u>Please!</u>

I am so sick about hearing about family values.
Most of us are in therapy because of our families.
I'm surprised you don't hear more calls
to 9-1-1— "Help me, I'm in a family,
get me outta here."

—Judy Carter

Clean Out Your Life

Just as you assessed your closet, take a look at your life. How many times a day do we tell our kids to clean up their messes? Stop and take a look at what's messy in your life. It may be your relationship with your sister, mother-in-law, coworker, friend, husband or ex—you fill in the blank. Whoever or whatever it is, do what you need to heal and GET OVER IT, MOVE ON, LET IT GO. Let go of anything weighing you down or holding you back. Speak to a professional who can help you work through your emotions. Really commit to solving the problem. It is impossible to be free and confident if you have negative energy surrounding you. Too often we clutter our minds with our own and other people's problems. It's time for a mental housecleaning. Hot Moms don't have time for drama, so clean out your life.

Let go of the way you thought your life was "supposed" to be and enjoy what it is. For a long time I attached myself pretty tightly to "the dream." Believe me, the dream did not include being a single mom. I struggled with this for a long time. I felt guilty about what I did wrong and angry about what my ex did wrong. I was mad at the world and mad at myself. How could I possibly be the best mom with all of that inner frustration? I couldn't. I wasted a lot of time blaming my ex and myself for my situation. Negative attitudes and energy create more negative attitudes and energy. So break the cycle. I did. Whatever you are holding on to in your life, drop it, let it go. Drama clutters up our homes as well as our minds. We all get figuratively trapped by our stuff. Letting go of stuff on a regular basis, be it physical or emotional, gives us breathing room and makes us feel fresh and new.

Woulda, Coulda, Shoulda— You Didn't, So Get Over It!

No one can change one second of the past, but mourning it can waste our present moments. Surrender to what is. Before we can change anything in our lives, we have to recognize that this is the way it is meant to be right now. Resisting what is happening in your life in the present only sets you up for frustration. When you stop resisting, your soul softens, you relax, you change your energy, you open yourself to positive things.

No two things can occupy the same space at the same time. In other words, either you can complain about your life or you can create the life you desire.

When we accept our circumstances we relax. It enables us to better see our next steps—what we need to do today to make a better tomorrow. Regret on some level is good in that it helps us gain wisdom and hopefully helps us to make better decisions in the future. So learn from your mistakes and let go. You are choosing and creating your life every day. Dwelling on the past will not do anything for you right now, so focus on where you are and where you want to be in the future, and make choices that will get you there. *What if* is a dangerous, no-win game that will only make you feel bad. The bottom line is that YOU are in control of your life right now. Teach your kids to take charge of their lives by taking charge of yours without looking back.

The movie *Sliding Doors*, starring Gwyneth Paltrow, portrays two versions of one woman's life side by side and shows how different her life would be had she caught the train one day instead of just missing it. If you have a serious case of the *what if*s, this is a good movie to rent.

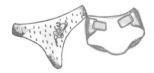

Tomorrow, Tomorrow,
I Love Ya, Tomorrow . . .

I know, I know: Tomorrow you will take that nap or enjoy yourself. It's always tomorrow, but life will never calm down long enough if we keep waiting for tomorrow. There will always be something vying for your attention—the phone, the kids. Life is always movement. Create little pleasures today. Every day. Now.

I can remember be impatient as a new mom, wanting and waiting for my son to say his first words, roll over, smile at me, walk, talk . . . hit all those milestones. But what is impatience? It's essentially rejection of the current moment as it is because something that we want to happen in a future moment hasn't yet occurred. What it does is deprive us of the pleasure of right now. Presence is about freedom, "living in the now," as many a New Age guru would say. Most of us, just like our kids, are more interested in what's happening next than what's happening now. LIVE NOW, in the present. It has been said that it's called the present because every day is a gift, so don't waste today thinking about the things you woulda, coulda, shoulda done.

> *Until you make peace with who you are, you will never be content with what you have.*
> —Doris Mortman

Worrying is another great thief of time. Like regret, worrying about the future robs us of the present moment. Living in and enjoying the moment—tuning in to all that is going on around you right now—is actually very simple, but it's not always easy for a busy mom to do. Tapping in to your senses is a good way to become more fully present. See, hear, smell, touch, taste, and *feel*. Most of us go about our days disconnected from the present moment. We live in the trance of our daily routine or habits. Whenever we do something the same way, over and over, it tends to become stale. We can easily and often get trapped in a rut and tune out.

Rut: (n) A fixed, usually boring, routine.

Just a small shift in the routine can jolt us to attention. With more attention comes more presence, so shake it up. Break the habit of your habits. Explore a new route to office or to school, rearrange your furniture, change your haircut, hike a different trail, try a new ice cream flavor, change your body wash to something really fragrant, try new foods, switch seats at the dinner table.

If you keep on doing what you've always done, you'll keep on getting what you've always got.
—W. L. Bateman

Little things can have a big impact. Make a conscious choice to vary one part of your routine each week.

All Bottled Up

Expressing your emotions is a release that detoxifies your body and soul. Any emotion becomes toxic when you bottle it up.

Suppressing something doesn't make it disappear.

Trying not to feel something is a form of resistance, and what you resist persists and gets stronger. Feel anger or frustration when it happens, with the kids. Experience the emotion. Allow it to be there and it will pass.

Once you start to feel emotionally free because you are no longer holding on, you won't get entangled in superfluous things—too many activities, possessions, buried feelings, and decisions that never get made. Just like with your clothes, you need to get rid of anything that is stale or not moving you forward. So get those feelings out, get rid of them so you can move on and move forward. Sometimes it's not the past but the daily pressures, like difficult kids, that are making you feel stressed and anxious. You need to find a release so you don't end up taking out your frustrations on your kids. I have a few suggestions in this chapter that will help you relax and unwind.

> *Wanna fly, you got to give up the shit that weighs you down.*
> —Toni Morrison,
> *Song of Solomon*

When you didn't have kids and you heard a mother yelling at her child, it's quite possible you thought to yourself, "I'll never yell at my kids like that." I did and I'm ashamed of my snap judgment . . . and also very sorry.

Because it's at that exact moment of snap judgment when the Gods of Irony, who know irony quite well, smile upon you and, lo and behold, you are given a child of your own who fights you on every little thing since they woke up at the crack of dawn. From not wanting to get dressed, to what they want to wear, to eating breakfast, what they want to play with, what they don't want to play with, getting into their car seat (where they amazingly become a human ironing board and not even Hercules himself can fold that little body into its seat), and everything in between.

And let's not forget the "I do." Not the fun and romantic "I promise to love you for the rest of my life, I do." The annoying, please god, don't let them say it . . . "I do dat Mummy." I know, I know. All the books say you should let them do it. Never mind you're going to be late. Never mind your schedule. Never mind it's going to add on an extra ten minutes when you're already ten minutes behind and you really don't have the time to let them master their zipper on this particular morning. Whatever.

Or even worse, you have two or three children fighting you on every single thing, or fighting with each other and wanting to do it all themselves. Again, I say, *whatever.* Sometimes things need to get done and we have neither the time nor the inclination to allow our little munchkins to do everything themselves. But we don't want to yell and have people judge us so we silently rage within.

But what are we to do about this silent rage, this silent screaming? I don't know. Maybe we can start by acknowledging that it's something that does happen; that at some point in our parenting career, many mothers (and fathers) feel it. We are human; we make mistakes. Screaming at our children isn't the answer but neither is keeping it inside where it's festering and affecting our health. Maybe we can stop judging other parents when they have a bad moment. Maybe when you see a parent losing it, you can go over and offer help or a sympathetic ear. And maybe, just maybe . . . in return, when you have a bad moment, they will do the same for you.

—Sharon DeVellis, Hot Mom of two boys, editor of YummyMummyClub.ca

Breed 'Em and Weep

I know it may seem a little ironic to suggest letting out a good cry when most of your time as a mom is spent trying to soothe your kids when they bawl. Crying is cathartic. Crying isn't just for people who have been through something traumatic or who are severely depressed. Most of us accumulate little conflicts or resentments or stresses during the day or week, and they can add up. Sometimes a good cry can really make you feel better. Our tears carry with them toxins and chemicals that build up from stress and remove them from our bodies. Not crying can actually increase stress and blood pressure. There is a scientific reason crying makes us feel better. One thing it does is lower our manganese levels. Overexposure to manganese can cause anxiety, fatigue, irritability, aggression, and nervousness.

> *If we had no winter the spring would not be so pleasant; if we did not sometimes taste of adversity, prosperity would not be so welcome.*
>
> —Anne Bradstreet

I had a good cry last week. I was feeling really overwhelmed with deadlines, this book, the magazines, and a few other Hot Moms Club projects. There was so much pressure, which was mixed with guilt for not being able to spend as much time with my son as I finished all of this up. I was doing a good job of putting on a brave face, but when I saw that Free Hugs Campaign video that was going around the Internet, I just lost it. I started crying, then sobbing. I'd seen the video before; it is so touching and always gets me teared up. But this time I think it served as a release for all that I had been stressed about and holding in. I felt infinitely better afterward. So if you haven't had a good therapeutic cry in a while, go for it. Surrendering to emotions doesn't mean being defeated by them. It's the difference between riding the wave and fighting it.

Emotional pain often means that you are getting stronger and that things are improving—the same way a house is in complete disarray during a renovation. You remind yourself that all of the mess will lead to a more beautiful home, and the same is true with the emotional turmoil.

Hug It Out

By now, more than 62 million people have watched the Free Hugs Campaign video on YouTube, if you haven't yet, it is worth Googling. Hugs have warm and fuzzy associations, and for good reason. Hugs are so powerful because humans thrive on being touched. The simple act of hugging can lift a person's spirits and make her feel connected. There is nothing like a warm, hearty hug from someone you care about. A well-placed hug can defuse emotions, help to bridge differences, and remind us that we matter. Don't wait until it's bedtime to hug your kids; find fun excuses to hug them throughout the day. Give your husband a solid, warm hug before he goes to work. Hug your friends when you meet. Encourage your kids to hug each other after they get in an argument. While hugging may not solve all of your problems, it will make you as well as the recipient feel better, and any peaceful, loving act is certainly a step in the correct direction.

A hug is like a boomerang—you get it back right away.
—Bil Keane, *Family Circus*

A hug is a smile with arms, a laugh with a stronger grip.
—Terri Guillemets

Arm ourselves for war? No! All the arms we need are for hugging.
—Unknown

Oh, I love hugging. I wish I was an octopus so I could hug ten people at a time.
—Drew Barrymore

Hugging is practically perfect: There are no movable parts, no batteries to replace, no periodic check-ups, has low energy consumption, high energy yield, is inflation-proof, non-fattening, no monthly payments, no insurance requirements, is theft-proof, non-taxable, non-polluting, and is, of course, fully returnable.

—Sharon Lindsey

Nearly everyone has been hurt at some point by the actions or words of another. Some of the world's most famous people talk about the power of forgiveness. We continually see stories of remarkable forgiveness on the news or read about them in history books. But practicing forgiveness may be tougher than getting a set of triplets to bed at night. It's hard because we often want to satisfy our need for justice, and forgiving feels almost like we are letting the person who hurt us off the hook. Holding on to anger can feel like a sort of punishment for them. Let go of your grudges. LET THEM GO. This isn't always simple, but it's necessary. The more confident and secure you are with yourself, the easier this will be. Hot Moms don't have time for grudges. Realize that the hate you feel toward an enemy

Forgive: (v) 1. To excuse fault or an offense.
2. To renounce anger or resentment.
The Aramaic word for "forgive" literally means "to untie."

or someone who has hurt you does not harm them at all. Nelson Mandela once said, "Resentment is like drinking poison and then hoping it will kill your enemies."

It's good to remember that your own peace and calm is not possible without forgiveness. When we are hurt by someone we love and trust, it can make us confused, angry, and really sad. If you dwell on these feelings or on the hurtful events, the grudge becomes resentment and hostility. Don't let the negative feelings crowd out the positive ones, and don't be engulfed by your own bitterness or sense of justice. If you are holding a grudge or resentment or harboring ill will, forgive. You owe it to your children to forgive. When you hold anger inside, it often leaks out against people, even your kids, who have done nothing to deserve it. You will bring anger and bitterness into every relationship whether you realize it or not. It can color your experiences in life and ruin your ability to truly feel the joy in each moment. Start by forgiving yourself; no one is perfect (aside from maybe David Beckham). We are all growing and learning everyday. There is enormous

> *Forgiveness is the scent of the flower that clings fast to the heel that crushed it.*
> —Mark Twain

> *Always forgive your enemies; nothing annoys them so much.*
> —Oscar Wilde

> *He who is devoid of the power to forgive is devoid of the power to love.*
> —Martin Luther King Jr.

healing and power in forgiveness. But it takes guts. It's not easy and it is more difficult if the person has not apologized.

Forgive without expecting reconciliation. You are doing this for you and your kids. Peace and calm are built on the decisions we make and the actions we take in the small moments of our lives. Deciding to forgive is one more way of creating peace. It is a way of freeing yourself from that person or situation and negativity. You may have been wronged and your feelings may be perfectly justified, but it is still up to you to choose to forgive and bring an end to your upset. It is impossible to forgive someone if you still feel angry with them.

> *Hate is like an acid. It destroys the vessel in which it is stored.*
> —Ann Landers

So let out all of your emotions. Express how you feel. Write a letter (which you won't send) or scream out the window or cry into a pillow; just get it out from inside of you. Then stop telling the story. Repeating the wrong to anyone who will listen only magnifies its significance in your life and glues it to you. While you are at it, forgive yourself; no one is the perfect mom, and we all have bad days. Try to learn from it and let it go. The more you pay attention to negativity, the more influence you give it. What you are you summon toward you. Anger attracts anger, fear attracts fear, kindness attracts kindness, love attracts love. What emotions dominate you? Gratitude, love, excitement, anger, resentment, exhaustion?

It is said that resentment becomes a habit and that habits in general take about thirty days to change. A technique to help you lessen resentment and build com-passion for a particular person or situation is to close your eyes for ten or fifteen seconds and picture the person who has hurt or angered you. Let all your feel-ings come up to the surface. Your heart may start to race and you may feel a tightening and tension through-out your entire body—that's normal. Now take a few long, deep breaths. Release the image and bring a new picture to your mind, of someone you love or a place or memory that makes you feel happy. Allow yourself to be filled with positive feelings. Hold this for a minute or so. Now imagine the person you are angry with again, but let the good feelings pro-tect you. The reason you do this is to break the pattern of stress reactions that you are programmed to feel when you think of the person who has wronged you. If you fill your heart with positive feel-ings when you think of them, over time (again, it takes about thirty days to fully change a habit) it will literally change your mental and physical reactions. They will lose their power over you—you will be reprogrammed. The same is true with sending him or her good wishes; for some reason, whatever we wish on others seems to have a rebound effect. So the next time you think of the person who has upset you, wish them well; note that they are in need of a blessing and compassion. At first it will feel contrived, but eventually the technique forces your mind to overcome the discrepancy between hating and acting with compassion. And eventually you will really feel this way.

> *The weak can never forgive. Forgiveness is the attribute of the strong.*
> —Gandhi

Forgiving doesn't mean forgetting or even returning that person to their former status in our lives. It is not acceptance of wrong behavior, as painful memories can often protect us from future hurts. Forgiving means we have moved on and healed from the hurt that has been done to us, and we refuse to continue to be its victim.

This is also a great technique to teach a child who's upset with her brother for eating the last cherry Popsicle or for breaking her favorite doll carriage.

Happily Ever After Divorce

Whether you chose to leave the marriage, or that no-good rat bastard ex of yours—Anyway . . . work through your issues. Don't make things harder on your kids by fighting. This seems obvious, but don't say anything negative about their dad in front of them. Even if it's true, it is hurtful to your children to hear that. Love your kids more than you hate each other. Make every effort to work through any pain or resentment.

Ah, yes, "divorce" . . . from the Latin word meaning "to rip out a man's genitals through his wallet."
—Robin Williams

Holding on to anger is like grasping a hot coal with the intent of throwing it at someone else; you are the one getting burned.
—The Buddha

Some of you mistakenly feel that because your marriage ended, you're at a disadvantage. Ladies, nothing could be further from the truth. Think of all the invaluable experience: You know what it takes to make a relationship work, and what will make it crash and burn; you are better able to weed out the losers; you know all the signs, good and bad, so you will be able to assess if he will be a good husband. At least you tried—at least someone picked you. Your stock is higher because you've been picked. Men register this in their minds whether consciously or subconsciously. Remember, you're not desperate. You know that, yes, you can recover from heartbreak, and no, he's not the last man on earth. Don't waste one more second of your time or your youth on someone who has rejected you. Know it is better to be alone and happy than in a crappy relationship.

—Patti Stanger,
star and executive producer of
The Millionaire Matchmaker

Being divorced is like being hit by a Mack truck. If you live through it, you start looking very carefully to the right and to the left.
—Jean Kerr

Be Brave

I have made many mistakes, and I make new ones every day, but I've quit concentrating on them and started learning from them. One of the biggest mistakes I made was being afraid to take a chance and staying in a relationship when my spirit knew it was time to leave. I have learned that if you let your soul guide you and you bring your confidence along, you'll always land on your feet. The hardest part is deciding to do it. So while you are cleaning out your life, don't forget to toss away all of your insecurities and your fears. Hot Moms are bold, Hot Moms know who they are, and they don't let anyone put them down or discourage them. Hot Moms aren't afraid to go after what they need and want in life. Leaving a great, well-paying job to start the Hot Moms Club was a huge leap of faith for me, and it was scary at times. Uncertainty always is. We make decisions based on either love or fear—fear of never meeting anyone else, fear of failure, etc. I chose to be brave and not let my fears consume me, to make my decisions based on my passions and loves, and so far everything has worked out the way I had hoped and envisioned. It wasn't always an easy path, but it was the right path for me.

Your Inner Circle, Square, and Triangle

Just like with your closet, keep only the people and relationships that make you feel good. It is so important to surround yourself with people who are positive and fun. You become who they are, so make room in your life for wise souls and people who inspire you. You wouldn't encourage your kids to hang around with anyone who wasn't nice to them or good for them; make sure the people closest to you have traits and characteristics that motivate you and propel you forward. Our children mimic our relationships and how we deal with them. Decide what and who needs to be in your life and make room for what and who you want.

Also, just as you might add a colorful new piece to your wardrobe, don't be afraid to befriend someone colorful and new. Life is an endless opportunity to learn. Letting go of old feelings and habits allows you to open yourself up to new people and new experiences.

People Politics

It is impossible to please or get along with everyone all the time. We all strive to maintain balance and personal power in our relationships. You are going to encounter difficult people or people whose personalities clash with your own. Difficult people come in every conceivable variety. It is all too easy to let emotions lead the way and take their behavior personally, but try hard not to. Their behavior is habitual and likely affects most people they come into contact with. A difficult person's attitude or underlying message is often, "Unless you agree with me and go along, you'll regret it." Usually we can't resist getting riled up in our own defense. Don't try to appease them; difficult people have an insatiable appetite for more. And don't try to change them. You can't control others, but you can control yourself and your actions.

> If you don't have enemies, you don't have character.
> —Paul Newman

Snipers

Watch out for what I like to call snipers—people who attack in subtle ways like taking potshots, using sarcasm, and making jokes at others' expense.

Most people who are mean, defensive, or scheming are that way because they are hurting or angry inside. Anger stems from hurt. Knowing this can help you to respond with compassion. It can be especially hard as mothers to control the "mama bear" urge to protect when someone insults or harms our child or someone we care about.

> Hurting people hurt people.
> —Joyce Meyer

As an Italian from Jersey, it is hard for me to bite my

tongue sometimes. It is something I have to work on. I get it from my mother. I remember one incident in high school during a track meet on a particularly warm day. I had just run a race and hit one of my best times. But afterward I felt sick and I was vomiting in a garbage can. Some boys walked by, and one said, "Ewww, that's gross!" Without missing a beat, my mom yelled, "Yeah? Well, what do you expect? *She saw your face!*" His friends started laughing at him for getting dissed by a mom.

Difficult people rely on familiar tactics to rattle or intimidate you. They count on you to respond in a predictable way. Try not to fall into their trap. Ease the situation by staying calm. Ask, "When you say that, what are you really trying to say?"

> *If you hear that someone is speaking ill of you, instead of trying to defend yourself, you should say, "He obviously doesn't know me very well, since there are so many other faults he could have mentioned."*
> —Epictetus

Hot Mom Commitment: Commit to assessing your closet and your life; they work in tandem. Commit to letting go of the old, whether it's old clothes, old habits, or old grudges, or negative people, and invite new, wonderful people and situations into your life. And try to control your responses to the difficult people you can't avoid.

Mothers relate to other mothers. As you start to see other moms in a new light, you may also gain insight into, and newfound appreciation for, your own mother. Whether you are already the best of friends or haven't spoken in years, your relationship will inevitably change. Having a child of your own will bond you to your mom in ways that you never imagined. As your child grows you will understand why she did the things she did or said the things she said, why she worried so much, or why she is so attached to you and invested in your life choices. As a parent you may plan to be just like your mom or you may strive to be the opposite. The great thing is that no matter how you were raised, you get to decide the type of parent you want to be.

We live in a society that is conditioned to blame problems in our lives on what our parents did or didn't do to us growing up. Maybe they were around too much and controlled and smothered you or weren't around enough and left you with commitment issues. Who knows. There is no doubt that our upbringings have a strong impact on who we are today and how we parent. You can dwell on your past or you can make it work for you. Sometimes looking back can help us to move forward. We are conditioned by the time we are toddlers, when lifelong patterns are imprinted into our brains. Your state of mind has just as much influence on your kids as your parents' did on you. In the first year of your baby's life their little brains learn how to feel, behave, and think based on the influences in the home. You owe it to your children to create a loving, happy environment, and that starts with you. Letting go is ironically the only way to get it together. Don't be a victim of what did or didn't happen to you growing up. You get to decide the type of parent you want to be now.

Until You've Walked a Mile in Their Robeez

I was hiking with my son once when he was four or five years old, and halfway through our hike he was running (when I told him not to) and of course he tripped and skinned his knees and hands. We were in the dead middle of the trail and had a bit to go to get to the car. As much as I tried to comfort him, he was crying about how much it hurt and how he needed me to carry him. Admittedly I was feeling frazzled and anxious, and I could barely lift him and walk uphill. Any mom knows there is nothing more unnerving than hearing her child cry—knowing he was in pain and not being able to do anything about it made me feel helpless and upset myself. At one point I stopped and told him in a firm voice that he was being dramatic and had to stop crying, that we were almost finished and I would soon be able to take care of him. Wouldn't you know it, not even a few steps later I tripped, fell, and skinned my knee and hand. I hadn't done that since I was a little girl. And WOW, did it hurt, and boy, did it sting. I had forgotten how painful it was—and my son's wounds were much worse than mine. I immediately held and kissed him. As painful as it was, I needed that experience at that moment so I could truly empathize with him. In general as a mom, I was always quick with a Band-Aid and a feel-better kiss, but from that time on my compassion for boo-boos came from a different place: from fresh remembering.

> We see the world
> not as it is,
> but as we are.
> —Stephen Covey

Until we have experienced something we really don't know how it feels. We can sympathize, but we don't really know until we are in that position how we would react. So go easy on people.

A new attitude can change the dynamic of a relationship.

One fall, at a parent-teacher conference with the father of a boy I'd had many problems with all year, I poured out a list of his son's many infractions. The father looked at me puzzled and said, "This is strange, because my son told me you're his favorite teacher."

I began thinking, This poor boy, he has no idea how to show his feelings. He must not understand how to show appreciation. For the remainder of the school year I looked at the student differently. I was more patient, kind, and understanding. In turn he became kind and understanding. At the end of the year he brought me a little gift and thanked me for a great year. He then told me that he was so surprised when his dad returned from fall conferences and told him that he was my favorite student. Our relationship would have never healed if it were not for one very smart parent.

—Hilary Probst,
Arizona teacher and Hot Mom of two

Take the Opposite View

Joy Bergin and I started a Hot Moms Club talk radio show on XM, and much of it is about hot topics. Joy is often very opinionated and she is not shy about expressing herself. Sometimes I agree with her, and sometimes for the sake of argument I have to take an opposite viewpoint. It's refreshing to see things and to argue from a slightly different perspective. So next time you are examining a situation, look at it from all perspectives, take a different view, and see if it helps.

It's hard sometimes to put ourselves in our kids' shoes, to really understand them or look at things through their eyes. Every day they are learning, growing, trying, failing, trying again . . . When I was studying to become a teacher, I had a professor who taught us that whenever we were getting frustrated with our students because they weren't "getting" a concept or understanding what we were trying to teach, we should pick up a pencil and try to write with our opposite hand. She said that this was what it feels like for students. It helped us understand that it can be awkward and frustrating to learn new things, it was a great way to help us exercise compassion. The same principle can be applied to our children, toddlers through teens, who are figuratively learning to write with the opposite hand every day.

Bad Days: It's Okay to Have Them

You are flawed, I'm flawed, we all are. You are not perfect, I am not perfect, and we never will be—and you know what? It's okay. It's okay to not always be okay. We're human, and some days we may not want to turn that frown upside down. You are going to have some days when you feel really good and some days when you feel blah or upset about something. Don't fight it; feel it, be pissed off, be bummed—but move on; don't wallow. Give yourself space to feel your emotions. Try not to take it out on your kids. But feel what you are feeling. It's okay to have a bad day or even a bad week, just don't make a habit out of it or before you know it you will have a bad life. You can restart your day anytime you want. You don't have to wait till morning to shift your mood if you feel you just can't stand one more stinkin' minute of the bad day.

> *Some days you're a bug, some days you're a windshield.*
> —Price Cobb

A few weeks ago, I arrived at the airport for my six a.m. flight only to find they had no record of me. An experienced traveler, I had checked in online and had my confirmation number. Well, it turned out that I had booked the tickets in the opposite direction: I was on a six a.m. flight *to* L.A., not *from* L.A., and vice versa for the return. How could I have done that? To make matters

> *I know the Lord will help—but help me, Lord, until You help.*
> —Hasidic prayer

worse, my son was with me. Fortunately they had seats on the next flight (two hours later), but the $300 in change fees did not have me feeling so grateful. I was upset with myself for making that error. When we got to the gate I took a few deep breaths and tried to turn it around. It was a lesson in going slow, in taking my time and lightening my load so that I didn't make simple errors like that one. As moms we often take on too much. Bad days remind us that we are not superwoman and should stop trying to be.

> *Every day is a gift— even if it sucks.*
> —Sherry Hochman

Just Say No (to Everyone)

So much of our attention is focused outward, toward our kids and to the world. This chapter is about turning some of that attention inward, by healing and helping your spirit thrive. You have to make your light bright; otherwise, what do you have to shine on your children?

Women, especially mothers, need to feel validated, and it is all too easy to become addicted to the busyness. Saying *yes, yes, yes* creates an endless to-do list that never gets finished. It becomes harder and harder to relax, and so goes the

> *It's not so much all we actually have to do in any one week that kills us, it's thinking about all we have to do.*
> —Unknown

pattern. Saying yes to some activities outside the home is a good thing and important to your sanity; moms of young children especially need time to get out of the house to socialize and think about adult things besides coupons and how to keep breast-milk stains off a new blouse. But it is all about balance. Often as moms we take on too much. I am very guilty of this, because I have a hard time saying no.

"So how do you do it?" I asked a friend.

"Do what?" she replied.

"How do you say no?"

"I just say no," she answered.

It is really that simple. You shouldn't say yes to something just because you are capable of doing it. Really evaluate the time and emotional commitment and decide whether it is something you want to take on. Also, never say yes on the spot. Tell people you will get back to them after you have thought about it. If you decide you don't want to do something, acknowledge their request, address your limitations and how much you would love to partake, but . . . and then, if you can, offer alternatives. Stand your ground—be firm. We all like to get what we want, and we all experience rejection in some form or another. I have learned if you do say no, you don't have to offer up a ton of excuses; just say you have too much on your plate right now or that it doesn't fit into your schedule. Don't launch into guilt-ridden specifics of how much you would love to, but . . . You don't have to apologize for safeguarding your time.

Guilt is often connected to saying no to people. Our knee-jerk reaction is to acquiesce because it's simpler that way. When you say yes, you don't have to explain; the person responds favorably to your agreeing nature, and for a single moment you feel good—until you realize that you actually didn't want to agree in the first place.

—Christine Louise Hohlbaum,
author of *The Power of Slow*

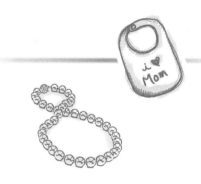

Monotasking

Hi, my name is Minsun and I am a multi-tasking addict. I justified my addiction for years because all the other cool moms were doing it. Peer pressure can be crushing in a society where a grown-up can't even justify a simple nap unless it is a "power nap." Not that I know anything about naps. As a stay-at-home mom to two boys, co-owner of a small business, tae kwon do practitioner training for my second-degree black belt, and freelance writer, not only is my plate full to overflowing, it's spinning in the air with many other plates.

Even though I really suck at multitasking, I still felt helplessly sucked in to doing it—until the day I hit rock bottom. It started off as a typically frantic morning when I spun around the house like a whirling dervish trying to get two kids and myself ready for the day. Since I had some meetings, I decided to be ambitious and try a sexy, smoky eye featured in some beauty magazine. Of course I was running late, so I choked down some cereal as I applied my makeup, checked e-mail, and tracked down my son's missing left shoe. When I got home that afternoon, I glanced in the mirror and gasped in horror. In all the chaos, I'd only managed to do one smoky eye and spent the whole day looking like a deranged, one-eyed panda. I hung my head in shame, only to notice that I was also still wearing my bedroom slippers. Talk about an epic multitasking fail.

I realized that I needed to detox from multitasking. So I resolved to quit cold turkey and try monotasking for a week. No easy feat in the Age of Distraction, when Facebook, texting, iPhones, laptops, and Twitter are ubiquitous gateway drugs for multitaskers like me. But recent studies show that multitasking is actually a myth because our brains simply aren't equipped for parallel processing. Although it may appear we are simultaneously accomplishing several tasks, multitaskers are merely switching back and forth between different tasks (or NOT, in my case) very quickly. So multitasking is actually a misnomer, and "high speed serial tasking" would be a more apt description. But it's not pithy enough to enter our lexicon anytime soon.

If multitasking is counterproductive and theoretically impossible, why am I still so addicted? Researchers at Stanford University confirmed this scientific irony in a recent study: The worse someone was at multitasking, the more they were compelled to do it. One theory is that the constant flow of data and busywork acts as a dopamine high, especially for a classic type A personality like myself. Another theory is that our multitasking ineptitude gets us stuck in a vicious cycle we can't extricate ourselves from.

So I modified the famous twelve-step program to address my own addiction. The first few steps to overcoming any sort of addiction are acknowledgment, acceptance, and making amends. Once I admitted to myself that I was a multitasking addict, I apologized to my kids for being frazzled and distracted, and resolved to change my ways.

Another important tenet is seeking help from others and a Higher Power. Although I'm not a particularly religious person, I do believe in God and pray. So I prayed fervently for Mary Poppins or even Julie Andrews to come to my rescue, which didn't happen. But what did happen was way more magical. My spiritual gurus and sponsors appeared— in the forms of my own two children. They are both veteran monotaskers and ascended masters at living in the moment. All I needed to do was follow their examples.

It's inspiring to watch my eight-year-old son, Jonah, methodically sifting through hundreds of tiny Lego pieces for hours to create a Star Wars X-wing fighter. Or to watch three-year-old Asher eat mac and cheese with complete and happy absorption. Meanwhile, I can't even take a bathroom break without dragging my laptop in with me (sorry, TMI). So I powered down, stepped away from my iPhone and my laptop, and went off the grid whenever I was with my kids. I told myself that I would check e-mails at appointed times and only answer or make urgent calls.

I had pretty strong withdrawal symptoms the first couple of days. Even taking a bathroom break made me anxious about e-mail I might've missed. But once I acknowledged those impulses, I saw them for what they were—mere impulses, not a necessity. Monotasking forced me to prioritize and I realized that most e-mails, calls, texts, and yes, Facebook feeds, really could wait until I could devote my undivided attention.

Even the tedious household task of conquering Mt. Washmore (aka laundry) became a meditative moment. Instead of anesthetizing myself with music or TV, I lit a scented candle and let my mind wander as I smoothed away wrinkles and folded clothing into tidy piles. I felt surprisingly calm and relaxed by this repetitious ritual once I accepted what I was doing and gave it my full attention.

By the end of the week, monotasking enabled me to live more in the moment—even the moments I'd rather not be having. Since I wasn't as strung-out and hopped up on stress by the end of the day, my entire family appreciated and benefited from a not-so-cranky and distracted mom. That's not to say I didn't cheat or fall off the wagon occasionally. Nothing turns my head like a brightly colored LED screen, and a relapse is only a seductive click and a scroll away. But life with my kids is far too fleeting to be twittered away, so I am taking it one moment, one task, and one over-scheduled day at a time.

—Minsun Park, blogger, SheKnows.com

Multitasking Is So Last Year

Getting upset, worried, stressed, and overscheduled is part of being a mom. Managing it and acknowledging it are important tools. Knowing how to calm yourself when you hit little bumps is crucial to your sanity and to being a Hot Mom.

Find time to take care of yourself. You are not the best mom unless you are the best YOU! Here are some ways to bring some Zen into your life on a daily and weekly basis.

Pamper: (v)
To indulge or gratify a desire; to treat with care or attention.

If pampering yourself means driving to drop off the videos at the store by yourself, you have a problem.

Groove

Music is powerful. It can invigorate your spirit and lift you up, or it can calm you and your kids down. Musical therapy has been an ancient tradition for centuries. Bells, drums, rattles, and such have been used to drive disease or despair from the body and soul. Music is said to reach beyond the barriers of our conscious minds. Rhythm reduces anxiety. Find music that moves your soul. There is music to fit your every mood. Sounds of the ocean waves, waterfalls, and other sounds from nature also have an incredible calming effect.

Create CDs for all occasions. I have a fun one for the car with songs my son loves and that put us both in a good mood. And I have a mix to calm us both down when we have had a long, busy day. Reconnect with music—play it, sing it, listen to; whatever you do, appreciate it and find what moves you most. (I used to listen to the radio when he was with me—the usual pop station, as we all do. I wouldn't pay much attention to the songs as I drove. Then one day I turned around to see my six-year-old bopping his head and singing Amy Winehouse's chorus, *"They tried to make me go to rehab and I said no, no, no."* That make me rethink radio. I respect moms who can do Radio Disney or kids' music in the car—my hat is off to you. But I can't do it in such a confined space for extended periods. So I create my own mixes of music I like that is appropriate for my son, too.)

Practice Gratitude

Be grateful, be glad you can see and are able to read this book, be thankful you are healthy and have healthy children; as crazy as they may make you sometimes, they are alive and playing. Gratitude opens our minds and hearts. Oprah talks about how keeping a gratitude journal has profoundly affected her life and the lives of those around her who keep them. She suggests taking a few minutes each morning when you wake up or at night when you go to bed (or both) to write down a few things you are grateful for. Entries can be as simple as, *I am grateful that the kids took naps today without complaint, I am grateful I spoke to my sister,* or *I am grateful to hear that bird chirping,* etc. We often have to remind ourselves how lucky we are. We take for granted simple conveniences and often overlook simple pleasures. Making gratitude a daily discipline will help start your day right.

If doing it daily seems like too much, you can also take a few minutes now and write down a long list of all the things and people you are grateful for in your life, then leave the list in your night table drawer or in your desk at work and look at it when you are feeling a little overwhelmed or frazzled. Add to

> *Gratitude opens our hearts and minds. It connects us with the present moment instantly.*
> —Unknown

> *Gratitude unlocks the fullness of life . . . Gratitude makes sense of our past, brings peace for today, and creates a vision for tomorrow.*
> —Melody Beattie

it when things happen for which you feel grateful. It is important not only to list and read these items but to actually FEEL grateful for them when you write or read your list. It's funny how our gratitude increases in direct proportion to how much we focus on it.

After writing this section I went back and made myself practice this exercise every day. At first I just thought I

> *I cried because I had no shoes, then I met a man who had no feet.*
> —paraphrased from *The Rose Garden*, by Saadi

would list a few things, but I was surprised that once I started I couldn't stop. I would (and still do) just get thinking of things to be thankful for, big and small, and I had to go on to the next page before I finally stopped myself. What I found was that throughout the day, and every day now, I look at things and think, I am so grateful for this moment, or this memory, whether it's tea and laughter with friends, an amazing dessert at a new restaurant, a sunny day, that my plane landed safely, or that my son caught the ball for a touchdown in his game and felt proud of himself. You get the point. And I strongly, deeply encourage you, even beg you, to trust me

> *The test of all happiness is gratitude.*
> —G. K. Chesterton

on this and do the same. Start your gratitude journal now. Don't put it off. Frankly, you will not be the same person one month from now after giving thanks each day for the wonderful abundance you already have in your life. It is said that the more you have and are grateful for, the more you will be given. It's the law of attraction. If that isn't motivation, I don't know what is. As simple a task as this is, it is amazing how much it helps you to see your world differently.

The website ButterBeeHappy.com is a free virtual online gratitude journal. It allows you to look for postings from people whose happy thoughts are similar to yours. Users say it reinforces their own good feelings. They also have a Happiness Hotline on which you can record an upbeat message for an online podcast.

Any blank book or piece of paper will do, so there is no excuse! For the long term, try a journal that excites you and invites you in. It has been said that it is the smallest details that make life worth savoring. So pick a journal that expresses your personality and style.

Journaling is something entirely different from the gratitude exercise, but it seems appropriate to bring up here. Maybe it's because I write every day, whether for a magazine or blog or for a book, but I admit I rarely keep a journal consistently. I know how much I love going back and reading the musings of my crazy mind when I stumble upon an old journal, and immediately I start to write again. But then, sure enough, after a few days or a week or two I forget or life gets too busy. But feeling like it is important to practice what I say, I decided to start again, and I can tell you, it is so freeing. The key is to write anything—don't edit in any way. No matter how silly or strange, let the words come. In the beginning you may find yourself complaining a bit. That's normal; it's your way of releasing some frustrations and finding solutions. A mentor once told me I shouldn't get a fancy journal to start out with, because if it was too pretty I would feel pressure to make it perfect inside, too. So grab a spiral notebook and go for it. This is also a great practice for your kids. I started my son on a journal last year and he has to write in it for ten minutes every day he is with me. I can't wait for the day that we can read it together. Hopefully he will find it amusing enough to share with me, and if not, I hope it brings him some laughs as he looks back, and I hope it starts him on this daily tradition of writing his feelings and thoughts.

Once you are feeling grateful, spread the happy feelings. Tell your kids how wonderful it is to spend time with them. Sharing and acknowledging wonderful memories is a powerful tool to prolong the joy and sustain the emotion. How we think and what we do can intensify the best moments in our lives. So tune in to the small stuff, give thanks, and spread the love.

A friend of mine was recently griping about something that was going on with her ex-husband, and since I was writing this section of the book, I suggested she write down all of the positive things about her situation: she receives enough child support so that she doesn't have to work (unlike many of the hard working single moms I know), he is an involved dad, she has a every other weekend free to go on trips or spend with friends. And although she smirked as she indulged me, she said afterward that writing down and focusing on all of the good made her feel a ton better, and she actually shared this gratitude with him. Their relationship has improved dramatically. It is amazing how a simple adjustment in your attitude can make a huge impact in your everyday life. So try it. What are you grateful for?

> *With a pencil and paper I could revise the world.*
> —Alison Lurie

Breathe

Breath is the essence of life. Taking time to regulate your breathing enhances your physical, emotional, and spiritual well-being. Your breathing integrates the many layers of your life. It is the key to health and happiness.

Take a deep breath and hold it. Notice the discomfort that builds as you resist your natural impulses to exhale. When it's too uncomfortable, release your breath and notice the immediate relief that sweeps over you. Holding on to anything when it is time to let go creates stress and discomfort in your body and mind.

Now completely empty your lungs and do not inhale. Pay attention to the discomfort that develops when you resist something you are meant to allow into your life. Breathing is a natural process of absorbing what we need and eliminating what we don't. Each day take time to exhale some stress and invite in laughter and tranquility. When you find yourself overwhelmed, take some of that age-old advice and *just breathe*.

A great exercise when you need a little sanctity is to make sure you are breathing deep enough so you can hear your inhales and your exhales. Focus on that sound—this is the breath we use in yoga that helps us through some of the more challenging poses. It forces you to be present in the moment and stay calm. I use this technique with my girls when they become frustrated. We count to

> five or ten while following the sound of our breath. Try it. It will work calming wonders for you and for them.
>
> —Elizabeth Blanchard,
> yoga instructor and Hot Mom of three

Spa Days

The airplane is like the spa for me. I actually look forward to travel because my phone doesn't ring. I can rest my eyes or relax into a book. It is a mini vacation in itself.

Pamper yourself at home—it sounds crazy, I know. Simply being able to go the bathroom without an audience half the time seems like a selfish indulgence.

But carve out a time each week, either when the kids are in bed or on those Saturday afternoons when they're at grandma's, and have your spa time. It is something you will look forward to all week.

First things first: Get yourself a spa "uniform." In order to feel truly pampered and glowing, you must be comfortable. I don't mean to get all Hugh Hefner on ya, but invest in a cozy robe—one that is soft and feels fabulous on, one that you never want to take off. While you are at it, get yourself a pair of snuggly slippers. You can't feel serene if you are not comfortable.

Bath Time Is Not Just for Kids

One of the most pampering pleasures in life is soaking in a luxurious, pleasantly scented bath. Baths increase body circulation and relax muscles. Soaking in water cleanses more than just your body; it unwinds and rejuvenates your spirit and soul. Your muscles loosen up in the warmth of the water as it works its calming miracles. It is easier than you think to create a gourmet bath experience. Create a box of your spa items that you can whip out when you have the alone time. Scented candles create a powerful mood, day or night. Play your favorite soft music. Place a few drops of your favorite scented oils in the tub. Lavender before bed will help you sleep. Coconut oil helps lift your mood. Use citrus for when you are feeling ill and Epsom salts if your back is aching.

Add a little bubbly . . . a bubble bath will remind you of your childhood and can make your feel frivolous and spoiled. Dropping flower petals or flower tops into the bath can also make it extra special. Have the kids help you gather some from your yard or on a walk and add a few to their baths, too. To appeal to all of your senses, add a few drops of color to your bath, as it is said that colors affect your mood. Eau LaLa and Crayola make nontoxic colorful bath tints and tablets that do not stain, all less than ten dollars. Blues and greens create a sense of tranquility. Pink also relaxes you. Purple will make you feel comforted and creative. Yellow recharges and energizes you. Red and orange arouse passion and excitement. (This is fun for the kids, too—I would suggest blue and green for them, though!)

Carve out time to take a luscious bath when the kids are in bed. Enlist the help of your hubby or hire a sitter to take the kids out to the movies or bowling or something else fun once a week so you get some relaxation time in your own home.

Aromatherapy

Our sense of smell is closely linked to neurotransmitters in our brains. When we inhale a scent, it triggers chemical reactions that affect our mood and emotions. Essential oils, through either a massage or bath, penetrate the epidermis, stimulating the lymph system, entering the bloodstream, and contributing to a state of well-being. Check out your local health food store for natural and organic essential oils. Essential oils are not the same as perfumes or artificially created fragrances; they come from real plants and are the most potent and concentrated extracts from various parts of flowers, fruits, leaves, spices, roots, and woods. They have therapeutic psychological and physical benefits. Mint, lavender, and chamomile seem to be popular with moms because they have a calming effect. Once you find a scent you like, place a few drops of oil in your garbage can, kitchen drain, and vacuum bag filter—or use a diffuser to keep a room in a blissful state. Remember, though: Some essential oils are powerful, so they should be diluted with water and never applied directly to the skin or swallowed. Make sure to follow all of the manufacturer's directions.

Dr. Kurt Schnaubelt is an industry leader in aromatherapy. His site OriginalSwissAromatics.com has a top selection of essential oils and therapeutic blends.

Baby Massage

When Kourtney Kardashian posted photos on her blog of her baby, Mason, getting a pampering massage, many eyes rolled. While a standing appointment for your teething tot at Burke Williams may be a bit over the top, creating an in-home spa is beneficial and fun for both you and your little one. Just some of the advantages of the baby rub down: It improves circulation, helps enhance the immune system, stimulates neurological development, helps babies to sleep more deeply, relaxes and calms them, helps with gas and colic, and improves their general well-being. Massage is ideal for infant-parent bonding, provides one-on-one quiet time, and encourages preverbal communication between parent and child. This is also a great way for parents to relax and unwind. And it can be a nice bonding ritual to involve dad. There are specific techniques for properly massaging your baby. Look for classes in your area and instructional clips and videos online.

Attitude: Try to Keep a Positive One

One of the best ways to get through life's bumps and to pamper yourself is to keep a positive attitude. It has been said that that the world is our mirror; it reflects back at us what we put out there. Energy attracts like energy; it makes sense that positivity attracts positive results and lucky coincidences. You

> The glass is always half empty. And cracked. And I just cut my lip on it. And chipped my tooth.
> —Janeane Garofalo

owe it to your children to be at your happiest and best, and they will return the favor by being at their best.

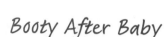

Five

Booty After Baby

When I was pregnant, my doctor told me to exercise more than I normally would. Uh, that would be a coma.

—Stephanie Blum, comedian and Hot Mom of three

When we become moms, it is more important than ever to take care of our bodies. Why? Taking care of your body affects your mood, your energy, and your physical and mental health. I know getting back into shape can feel like a hard commitment when you have a little one or little ones to look after, and at times it almost feels unattainable, but you really can do it. You only have one body, and if you look after it as though it is your shrine, it will look after you, keeping you young, energetic, and full of life.

This chapter is all about creating a healthy lifestyle. We owe it to our children to model good exercise and eating habits. Heck, we owe it to ourselves! Setting a good "workout ethic" for our kids with regular exercise is far and away one of the most important actions we can take as a parent. The obesity rate has risen 50 percent in the past fifty years in this country, and with all of the available technology today, we are raising a generation of couch potatoes and computer/ video gamers who don't exercise enough. It is up to us as parents to stop the cycle, first with ourselves and next with our kids, by setting a healthy example and new family routines.

> And baby makes three . . . additional dress sizes. Not only is having a baby a life-altering experience, it can be a clothes-altering experience as well. As anyone who has not graced the cover of *Sports Illustrated* will tell you, bathing suit shopping post-baby is worse than getting a Pap smear, a mammogram, and a bikini wax all at the same time.
>
> —Joanne Kimes,
> Hot Mom and author of *Dieting Sucks*

The Skinny on Post-Baby Bods

I know it can be hard to watch celebrity moms flaunt around in their swimsuits or skinny jeans just weeks after giving birth. (Thank you very much, Giselle.) Remember, celebrity moms have trainers, nutritionists, nannies, chefs, and full-time personal assistants—heck, their

I have flabby thighs, but fortunately my stomach covers them.
—Joan Rivers

personal assistants have personal assistants. And supermodels, well, they just have good genes. They also have a lot more pressure to get back in shape because their profession is looking good. And you thought it was bad having your hubby bug you about those few extra pounds. Imagine if you had tabloids following you around just waiting for a roll of post-baby flab to flop out from your jeans. Body slimmers and tummy toners are popular among Hollywood moms because they help get your stomach back to normal after pregnancy. (See chapter 3 for details on some of the Hot Moms Club's favorite brands.)

The Rumored C-Tuck

Rumor has it that to make sure their stretch marks never see the light of any flashbulbs, celebrity moms have tummy tucks immediately after their C-sections. Whether this is true or not, I don't know; not one celebrity I know would say (or at least would not admit it to me), but all of the doctors I spoke with recommend AGAINST this procedure, saying that it's dangerous; it's more surgery than is necessary, it puts you at a higher risk of infection, and it makes the healing process longer (when you should be bonding with your baby). Plus, they added that although it may sound convenient to have both procedures done at one time, the results aren't as effective. I was told that tummy tucks should not be performed until after the C-section has healed so that the doctor can see how the skin settles.

As with all elective surgery, do your research, get the facts, and talk to several doctors before making any decisions.

Kicking Back Versus Kicking Butt

You don't have to be a celebrity mom trying desperately to slim down for your steamy mock love scene with Will Ferrell to start taking fitness seriously. Staying healthy and fit is a lifelong commitment. As moms, our initial motivation might be to get our pre-preggo bods back, but there are other benefits. Regular exercise will alter you in ways you never thought. Making a commitment and sticking to it is a huge accomplishment in itself. The act of getting up and walking several times a week—actually doing it and keeping your promise—will enhance your self-esteem dramatically. There is a significant mental component to fitness. Try designing a program and setting goals so that you experience levels of achievement. A good exercise programs builds your spirit as well as your muscles. So start today. Figure out what you can do and how you can begin to work it into your schedule. Moms are multitasking goddesses. We ALWAYS make time

> *I don't exercise. If God had wanted me to bend over, He would have put diamonds on the floor.*
>
> —Joan Rivers

for the things we want and need to do. You just have to commit to making workouts a priority.

Get in Gear . . . Or Just Get Great Gear

Nothing motivates me to work out like cute workout clothes! It's all too easy to put off the track or the gym, and not too long ago I found myself in a slump. I was traveling a bunch and got so busy that my routine fell off. To get me in the mood again, I stopped by the Lululemon store near me (Lululemon.com) and it made me completely psyched to hit the track. Not only were the clothes trendy and comfortable, all the people working there were really helpful and excited about being active. They really made me feel like I was in good company, and I couldn't wait to go back and show them my progress.

I also picked up a pair of the hot new Reebok Easy-Tone shoes. They are specially designed to tone and strengthen key leg muscles with every step. The commercials say they help firm your butt and that is all I needed to hear. I have been using them and I am happy to report I feel and see a difference!

One of your best workout accessories is an iPod or MP3 player. Cut a soundtrack to get you pumped. This will make the workout more enjoyable and go by faster. Make sure choose upbeat songs—anything that makes you want to shake and move. Here are some of my favorite artists to work out with: Pink, Usher, Timbaland, Justin Timberlake, Black Eyed Peas, Rihanna, Beyoncé, U2, and Tina Turner.

"Alone" Comes from "ALL-ONE"

One of the most overlooked and underrated aspects of a mom's life is alone time. Find time for you and you alone. Find silence now and then. We need time when it's totally quiet to think, to feel, to regenerate, and to access our inner selves. Silent moments can be the most uncomfortable if we're used to all of the noise around and inside us. Wake up fifteen minutes early, before the rest of the family gets up. You can have your morning tea, stretch, and ease into your day before the craziness begins. A daily exercise routine is a great excuse for time to think and be alone. If that doesn't motivate, you I don't know what will!

Misery Loves Company

Find a workout buddy. Have a pal waiting for you, someone to gossip—I mean, *talk* with. Plus, if you make a commitment to someone, you are more likely to show and keep with your routine, encourage each other, make bets, whatever it takes to motivate you.

Invest in a trainer—most gyms offer a courtesy session. Having a trainer is really important in the beginning when you don't know what you are doing, and an expert will help get you working out properly and motivate you toward your goals.

BABY ON A BUDGET

Many celebrities hire trainers, and while their hourly rate may be out of your price range, most offer inexpensive DVDs that you can work out to.

Tracy Anderson (TracyAndersonMethod.com) has worked with Courteney Cox, Kate Hudson, and Gwyneth Paltrow.

Ramona Braganza (RamonaBraganza.com) has worked with Jessica Alba, Kate Beckinsale, Ashlee Simpson, and Halle Berry. She even has a twelve-week post-pregnancy workout, called 321 Baby Bulge Be Gone (321BabyBulgeBeGone.com).

Jennifer Cohen (JenniferCohen.com) not only whips brides into shape on the WB network, she is a regular fitness expert for the *Today* show. Her company is called No Gym Required; she believes you have all the tools you need to be fit right in your home.

Tracey Mallett (TraceyMallett.com) is an international fitness instructor, media personality, and author who has dozens of workout DVDs for all phases of post-baby life and all interest levels.

Quick tip: Buy health club memberships at the end of the month, or the end of the year, when salespeople are trying to make their quotas. You can bargain to get the best rate or discount. For example, try asking them to waive the initiation fee, to give you a free month, or to throw in free personal training sessions.

Celebrity Inspiration

Find a celebrity who looks amazing and has a body type similar to yours, or an athlete whose body you covet. Use that photo as inspiration when you are debating whether to skip a workout. Do want Michelle Obama's arms, Brooke Burke's tummy, or maybe Mary Louise Parker's legs? These moms prove you can look hot at any age no matter how many kids you have. Maybe it's not a celeb that inspires you but your goal weight from years ago or that dress you want to fit back into. Find a photo of someone (it can be yourself, pre-baby) that inspires you to get out that door and get moving!

Kelly Ripa is my body inspiration. She's a mom of three and she looks so lean and fit. But like many, Kelly found that fitness didn't always come naturally. She told *Fitness* magazine, "I didn't do it [exercise] in my 20s and I was like, it's too late to start now. I figured, I work in an industry where there's a stylist and a makeup artist—they'll make me look fine. But I began feeling tired—just playing in the park with my kids wore me down. I thought, 'Geez, I'm kind of young to be feeling this way.' So I started walking on a treadmill. Then I started jogging on a treadmill. Then I began jogging outside. Now I'm running outside, three to five miles, and taking toning classes. A month or two after I started working out, I wore a sleeveless turtleneck to work. Regis was like, 'Ripa, your arm muscles look incredible!' It was the first time anybody had ever said anything to me about my muscles. And because I am a vain person, that's all I needed to hear to stay with it!'"

Get Your "-ing" On

Cardio exercise is proven to burn fat. Running, jumping, biking, dancing, walking, hiking, rowing, skiing—these are all great workouts. Swimming is an ideal low-impact workout. So book it. Join a gym; take an aerobics, yoga, or dance class. You are never going to find the time, you just have to *make* the time. Just show up—just go to the gym. Tell yourself it will be an easy workout, or just start walking around the corner. Once your blood starts pumping, you will get into it.

> *My grandmother started walking five miles a day when she was sixty. She's ninety-seven now, and we don't know where the hell she is.*
> —Ellen DeGeneres

When you exercise, you have more energy, less stress, fewer weight problems, and generally a more positive attitude and outlook on life. People who don't exercise have every excuse in the world why they can't or won't find the time.

Cardio exercise is as essential to my daily routine as brushing my choppers. Even if it means that I am up before the paperboy in order to lace up my shoes and go for a run, then that is what I do. I have found that nothing does more for my sanity, *or vanity*, than some good, heart-pumping cardio. It reduces stress, gives me a shot of endorphins, and helps me manage my day—from high-pressure interviews to high-pressure temper tantrums. Remember, what bores your mind bores your body; you need variety, so keep an open mind and try something new.

I am a living example of how one can make positive improvements in their life not only to better themselves, but also to better the quality of life of those precious to them. I know about weight loss and what it takes to keep it off. I shed over seventy pounds after the birth of my second son. Being active has made me a better mother because I have a more positive outlook on parenting and life in general. I also have more energy. When people ask me what I do, I tell them I am an athlete. Normally the second question is, What sport? My answer: I am a mom. They look at me funny for a second, but then it sinks in. You can see the thought processing in their heads. Being a mom is a full-time job, with full-time physical demands, that is a never-ending marathon!

—Jennifer Nicole Lee, fitness expert, author, and Ms. Bikini America 2005

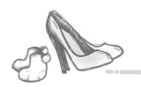

Dancing is a liberator of all things that hold us back.

—Angel Williams, fitness instructor

Zumba—Let's Get This Party Started!

Zumba is the latest craze. It is truly so much fun. Their tag line is "Ditch the Workout, Join the Party"— a fitness party, that is, and that is exactly what it feels like. Zumba fuses Latin rhythms and easy-to-follow moves. Their goal is to make you want to work out, make you love working out, and get you hooked. And it seems to be effective. I'm personally addicted, and apparently so are many other people; there are more than sixty thousand locations in 105 countries, millions of DVDs have been sold, and worldwide more than 7.5 million people participate in Zumba classes each week. Go to Zumba.com for more information and to find a class near you.

> *There's a territorial ritual to an aerobics class. I entered a class for the first time a few years ago and ended up where no one wanted to be . . . in the front row next to the mirror. It was three years before I could work my way to the back row.*
>
> —Erma Bombeck

Tai Chi

Tai Chi is an Asian martial art. It is a series of moves that flow from one to the other, with careful form at a gentle pace. It is one of the lowest-impact exercises you can find. Tai Chi improves balance, flexibility, and posture. Practicing Tai Chi for thirty to sixty minutes a day not only relaxes you but builds your muscles and burns calories. The Tai Chi Foundation (TaiChiFoundation .org) has locations in more than forty cities in seven countries.

Pilates

Pilates has hit the fitness mainstream. It encourages you to think about how you perform everyday movements. Using resistance apparatuses (small weighted balls, foam rollers, resistances bands, and others) it tones and balances and helps build strength without bulk. Pilates will not help with weight loss—you still need to work in a cardio routine—but it heightens your body awareness which in turn improves your overall agility, flexibility, and strength. It helps you ensure your body is working at its optimal level all the time.

Stand Tall

A fast, easy way to look great is to change your posture. Good posture instantly makes you appear slimmer. Sitting in front of a computer all day encourages our constant belly-bulging slump. Not only does good posture make you look taller and slimmer, it also improves your energy and digestion. When you slouch, less oxygen makes it to your muscles, and the blood flow to your gut is impaired, which can cause indigestion.

No Sweat

Did you know that we have more than two million sweat glands, covering almost every part of our body? Sitting in a sauna for thirty minutes produces the same amount of perspiration as running six miles. Activating your sweat glands requires energy; you can burn 300 to 500 calories after twenty to thirty minutes in a sauna. Saunas also help boost your immune system. If used properly and in moderation (twice a week for no more than a half an hour each session), saunas can be an effective method of health maintenance. (Talk to your doctor about what would be best for you.) Be sure to stay hydrated and drink lots of water before and after using a sauna.

As mothers, it is our job to provide a healthy platform from which our children can learn and grow. When they watch us fit exercise into our busy lives, they inadvertently mimic our actions and become healthy, active adolescents, then adults.

It really doesn't take much to incorporate fitness into our lives after baby. A walk in the park breathing fresh air benefits both mother and baby. Join one of the numerous child-friendly fitness programs that use baby for strength-training segments. Or take advantage of the daycare facility offered at most athletic clubs. Spend some quality time with family members strolling through your neighborhood after dinner, or find a group of stroller moms in your neighborhood who walk or run together.

—Andrea Vincent, founder of
See Mommy Run (SeeMommyRun.com)

Become a Babe with a Babe

Incorporate the kids into your fitness routine. So, you have a baby at home. Get creative and find a way to get those endorphins flowing every day. Walk with the kids, jump rope with them, swim, dance, run up and down the stairs, or run around after your three-year-old. Find out what interests you and *do it*! There is a form of release that fits into every schedule. If you don't have time to take a Zumba or hip-hop dance class, pop in a video and let the kids do it with you.

Take Stroller Strides

Lisa Druxman is the founder of Stroller Strides, a nationwide stroller workout for mom and baby. There are organized group walks for moms that combine intervals of body toning using the environment and your stroller. Mom achieves a total body workout and baby has fun. It's easier than a fitness class and it is all about mutual support and helping women succeed as new moms. With over twelve hundred locations nationwide, you can find a group near you (StrollerStrides.com).

HERE ARE A FEW OF LISA'S QUICK TIPS TO A GREAT STROLLER WORKOUT.*

✿ Start with an easy walk, gradually warming your body and muscles. The most common posture problem when pushing a stroller is hunching forward, so be sure to keep your shoulders back. (3–5 minutes)

✿ The squat is one of the best exercises for the lower body. Stand behind your stroller with the brake off, hand about shoulder width apart on the handlebar. Push your stroller out in front of you when you squat down, and pull it back as you pull yourself up into a standing position. (2 minutes)

✿ Try some interval training. Walk for 30 seconds as fast and hard as you can, then recover by slowing your pace for 30 seconds. Repeat until 3 minutes are up. (3 minutes)

✿ The lunge is one of the most effective exercises a woman can do to tone and strengthen her lower body. It's a compound exercise,

---

* Of course, always be sure your baby is strapped in safely before performing.

which means it works out a lot of muscles in just one move. Lunges work your quadriceps (front of your thigh) and hamstrings (back of your thigh) as well as your bottom. Lunge walk by taking really long lunge strides. (2 minutes)

❀ Power walk with your body tall and feet and knees facing forward. (3 minutes)

❀ Take time to stretch all of the body parts that you worked. This is a great time to pull your little one out of the stroller and stretch next to her. (5 minutes)

Say "Om"

Gwyneth Paltrow, Cindy Crawford, Madonna, and so many others have used yoga as a way to get their figures back. It is said that women who do yoga are more likely to have a healthy body image. Body image is the vision of yourself in your mind's eye. How we feel about our bodies is subjective, and unfortunately most people don't see themselves as they actually are. Yoga can help. Yoga in Sanskrit (the language of ancient India, where yoga originated) means "union," referring to the body, mind, and spirit.

Yoga involves stretching, poses, and postures, each with specific health benefits and varying levels of difficulty. Doing the poses in quick succession creates heat in the body. The poses are consistent across all types of yoga, but the approach to them varies depending on the type and the teacher.

Hatha describes any physical practice of yoga. It can be done by people of all ages and body types.

Power yoga involves performing a series of positions one after another in a more rapid fashion without resting in between.

Bikram or "hot" yoga is performed in a heated room to raise the body temperature and burn calories.

Yoga is so popular these days that it would be hard not to find a yoga class near you.

If you're looking for yoga gear, Manduka.com has high-quality mats, sleeves, slings, and towels, all in coordinating colors. They even have an eco line.

Gaiam (Gaiam.com) is one of the industry leaders in yoga gear and resources.

Set a good healthy example for your kids. My four-year-old daughter, Amber, loves doing Pilates and yoga with me. I caught her showing her friends some exercises. They were tickled pink trying to do a single leg stretch from Pilates and a downward dog in yoga. It was very funny to watch, and most importantly, they associated exercise with fun. This is excellent to instill at a young age.

—Tracey Mallett, fitness expert and author

So maybe you can't afford personal, one-on-one lessons with Mark Blanchard, Jennifer Lopez's personal yoga instructor, but you can order his complete instructional DVD set (MarkBlanchardsYoga.com), and if you live in Los Angeles you can take one of his classes or workshops—where you will surely bump into a celeb or two.

The Calming Power of Meditation

And while your endorphins are speeding up with your workouts, in your everyday routine I encourage you to slow down. Our modern lives move so fast; I hardly think humans were designed for it. It strains even those who thrive on multitasking. We haven't evolved to handle so much activity.

> I walk regularly for my soul and my body tags along.
> —Sarah Ban Breathnach

You must indulge your mind daily with peace and quiet. The activity going on in your brain is communicated to every cell in your body. When your mind is cluttered every cell tissue and organ is affected by that turbulence. You need to develop a method of calming and silencing your mind. This will generate peace and serenity throughout your entire body. Exercise quiets the mind and can be a great form of meditation.

> The Latin word for meditation, meditari (to think, to dwell, to exercise the mind), comes from the same root as the word mederi, which means "to heal."

Meditation is awareness, a

profound contemplation, thinking your mind into a deeper state of relaxation. When meditation is a part of your daily life you are less likely to overreact to everyday stresses. Meditation can help you temporarily escape a thought cycle and focus your attention. There are many ways to meditate, so don't let the word or idea scare you. Meditation is actually quite simple. You can do it right now, right where you are. But it is not always easy. Our minds do not like to be calmed. We often fluctuate among thoughts, stories, and memories in the space between two breaths. Our minds are like a puppy or your toddler; they can be willful but can be trained through gentle, persistent effort. The important thing is that you become still with yourself, that you become aware. Create an environment that lets your mind run free of thought. Steal a few minutes when the kids are napping, at lunch break, or early in the morning while the house is quiet. Breathe deeply and recharge. Think of something calming. Focus only on your breath; inhale and exhale. Find your touchstone. It is lifesaving to know how to rejuvenate yourself. You can meditate while sitting, listening to music, walking—walking is often said to be a moving meditation, a fitness of the spirit. A fifteen-minute walking meditation can take the edge off. Start by walking mindfully, at a normal brisk

Every time you meditate you are building a spiritual muscle. The more you use it, the stronger it gets. The energetic apparatus you build by meditating will absolutely change the way your life works.
—Diana Lang, author of *Opening to Meditation*

pace. After five minutes, slow your pace, and after another five minutes, slow your pace again so that you are walking slowly and deliberately. Focus your attention on each step you take. Be in the moment. If your mind starts to wander, bring it back.

Find what form of meditation works best for you, but in some way, every day, focus on restoring your peace of mind.

For as long as I can remember, long, hot showers have been my salvation. Whenever I feel anxious or stressed I find sanctuary under the steaming hot water. I didn't realize it at first, but this was my meditation. It was my time to be free of distractions and pressures. It was my time to be completely engrossed in the moment, the enjoyment of the water, and not in my thoughts. I have since polished and honed my skills and have found additional paths of peacefulness that don't run up my water bill or leave my skin dry!

> *I get totally absorbed and focused on riding my bike when I'm in the midst of it; it's my moving meditation. I find it brings me inner peace.*
>
> —Rochelle L'Italien, BMX mom

I often find myself completely overwhelmed. Yes, even me, a yoga teacher. So many times I have chosen not to ask for someone's help and instead added a tenth task to my to-do list. But as minutes, hours, days, and months pass, I am wising up. I think we can all wise up by asking. Ask for a lending hand, even if it isn't from someone you know but a higher source. Sometimes it takes courage to ask—to ask for strength, grace, a blessing, an ounce of compassion, or a pinch of peace.

In moments when we feel overwhelmed, it is simple to sit down and meditate for three to five minutes. Here's how: If you can, retreat into a quiet room. Sit on the floor and cross your legs Indian style or just sit in a chair. Bring your hands in front of you and cup them in front of your rib cage, your elbows at your sides. Your hands should be connected to each other as if you are making a big bowl with your hands. With your eyes closed, ask for simple grace. Allow your breath to be easy and smooth. Visualize everything you're asking for coming to you in spades, overflowing into the bowl in front of you. Allow yourself to move forward in this grace for the rest of the day and you might find it easier to let go a little more than usual. Maybe it's okay to do one or two things at a time and not three, or four, or five, or six . . . I think you get my drift.

—Anna Getty,
lifestyle expert, yoga instructor,
and Hot Mom of two

Attitude

You cannot succeed at any workout program without encouragement from your friends, family, and from yourself. Stay positive, stay focused on your goal, and visualize the outcome. It may be difficult at times, but keep on it and don't give up. You are a Hot Mom and nothing is going to stop you from achieving your goal.

Notice the difference between what happens when a man says to himself, "I have failed three times," and what happens when he says, "I am a failure."

—S. I. Hayakawa, former U.S. senator

I have missed more than nine thousand shots in my career. I've lost almost three hundred games; 26 times I have been trusted to take the game-winning shot and missed. I've failed over and over again in my life, and that is why I have succeeded.

—Michael Jordan

A group of frogs were hopping contentedly through the woods, going about their froggy business, when two of them fell into a deep pit. All of the other frogs gathered around the pit to see what could be done to help their companions. When they saw how deep the pit was, they agreed that it was hopeless and told the two frogs in the pit that they should prepare themselves for their fate, because they were as good as dead.

Unwilling to accept this terrible fate, the two frogs began to jump with all of their might. Some of the frogs shouted into the pit that it was hopeless, and that the two frogs wouldn't be in that situation if they had been more careful, more obedient to the froggy rules, and more responsible. The other frogs continued sorrowfully shouting that they should save their energy and give up, since they were already as good as dead.

The two frogs continued jumping with all their might, and after several hours of this, were quite weary. Finally, one of the frogs took heed to the calls of his fellow frogs. Exhausted, he quietly resolved himself to his fate, lay down at the bottom of the pit, and died.

The other frog continued to jump as hard as he could, although his body was wracked with pain and he was quite exhausted. Once again, his companions began yelling for him to accept his fate, stop the pain, and just die. The weary frog jumped harder and harder and, wonder of wonders, finally leaped so high that he sprang from the pit.

Amazed, the other frogs celebrated his freedom and then, gathering around him, asked, "Why did you continue jumping when we told you it was impossible?"

> The astonished frog explained to them that he was deaf, and as he saw their gestures and shouting, he thought they were cheering him on. What he had perceived as encouragement inspired him to try harder and to succeed against all odds.
>
> This simple story contains a powerful lesson: that there is both death and life in the power of our words. Your encouragement can lift others up and help them make it through the day. Your destructive words can cause deep wounds; they may be the weapons that destroy someone's desire to continue trying.
>
> —A fable

Recently my son and I visited the Exploratorium in San Francisco, where they have a booth that allows you to step in and see what it feels like to be cheered or booed, like sports figures on their home field or away. The booth also simulates what it would be like to give a speech to a standing ovation or a heckling crowd. It is remarkable how much impact encouragement can have on us. Create a support system for your exercise routine and be sure you are encouraging your kids. Whether it's for a soccer game or dance class, no matter what their interests, your enthusiasm and support will help them to excel at it.

What's Food Got to Do With It?

EVERYTHING! The quality of your life begins at the nourishment level. What you put inside your body absolutely affects how you look and feel on the outside. As moms, we sometimes focus so much on making sure our kids are fed, we often forget to eat ourselves. And no, a stolen bite or two of a peanut butter and jelly sandwich doesn't constitute a healthy lunch, even if you have four kids. As moms we run it all, and we can't afford to let our bodies get run down or get sick. We are teaching our kids the eating habits they will take with them through their whole lives.

Do You Diet?

There are literally hundreds of diets out there. Some are fads; some have been around for years. If you have found something that works for you, great! Natalie, on the Hot Moms Club team, loves Jenny Craig (as does Valerie Bertinelli—we all saw her in that bikini, and WOW). My ex-husband loves the Freshology food delivery service (as do Ricki Lake, Jennifer Lopez, and many other celebs). It's great if you are busy; the food comes fresh to your door each day, and the menu is prepared by chefs and nutritionists, so it's balanced and healthy (Freshology.com). You have to find the plan that is

> *What are the first three letters of "diet"? D-I-E.*
> —Mo'Nique, actress and comedian

> *I never worry about diets. The only carrots that interest me are the number you get in a diamond.*
>
> —Mae West

right for you. What works for me and what I believe in is a healthy lifestyle. If you adopt that, everything else will fall into place—your health, your weight, and your happiness.

The raw food diet gets a lot of hype, it's associated with celebrities including Demi Moore and Woody Harrelson. As you know, anything that is hot in Hollywood influences what we mere mortals do (carry around a small dog in a purse), wear (colorful rubber bracelets), or eat, hence the raw food diet. The raw food diet is really quite simple— you're not allowed to eat anything that's been cooked over 118 degrees. At first I thought that this was the ideal diet, since I know full well that Twinkies require no baking whatsoever. Unfortunately, there is another rule, that you must limit your food intake to fruits, vegetables, lean meats, nuts, and juice. That really sucked the fun right out of the diet for me, but if you are someone who enjoys a big plate of lawn, then go right ahead.

—Joanne Kimes,
Hot Mom and author of *Dieting Sucks*

A Cookie Makes It Feel Better

Emotional eating. We've all been there. You're feeling bummed about something and you go for comfort food. It's not your fault, really; it is likely a pattern started from your childhood. And it's true, comfort food can release endorphins that help you feel better, but it's temporary, and once it wears off, it's back to the original problem. As moms it is our natural reaction that when our kids get hurt or feel sad we want to make them feel happy, often by offering them a cookie or ice cream or some other treat. This creates a bad pattern where every time they feel upset, they think a candy or sweet will fix it. I am guilty of this myself. I picked up my son from school a few months ago, and he was really upset that his favorite friend was moving to another state. To cheer him up I took him to a fast food place, something I rarely do, and something he considers a big treat. He was all smiles, and I felt like Supermom for being able to save the day. A few weeks later I picked him up and he was upset about something else—and the first thing he said was, "Can we go to . . ." You guessed it: for fast food. That's when it hit me that I might be starting an unhealthy pattern. So the next time your kids feel sad, offer a hug or some one-on-one time instead of that cupcake.

Most of us eat for social reasons—eating to share good feelings or to hide bad ones. It is easy to forget the primary reason for eating, which is to nourish our bodies and provide ourselves with fuel. Eating should be fun, but eating healthy can be delicious.

Calories and Metabolism

Weight loss is a numbers game—you must burn more calories than you consume—but you must also eat the right foods. A calorie is a unit of energy. In general, adults need 1,200 to 2,000 calories a day for fuel; the amount your body needs varies, of course, depending on age, sex, weight, athletic level, and muscle mass. If you exceed the number of calories your body requires, you will gain weight. It takes an excess of approximately 3,500 calories to gain one pound of fat.

Empty calories are foods that contain little if any nutritional value. They are usually high in sugar or fat. They aren't satisfying and leave you hungry or craving more sugar. Empty calories translate into quick weight gain. Chips, cupcakes, candy bars, hard candies, soda, pie, cheese balls—all of these are examples of empty calories.

Negative-calorie foods are foods that are said to have some calories, but they require more calories to digest than the food contains. These foods are harder for the body to break down and process, so the body has to work harder to extract the calories, giving them a natural fat-burning advantage. Most fruit like apples, grapefruit, strawberry, blueberries, tomato, mango, papaya, raspberries fall into this category. Vegetables including celery, onion, spinach, zucchini, cucumber, carrot, broccoli, green beans are also considered negative-calorie foods.

Metabolism comes from the Greek word *metabole*, which means "change." It's how your body changes food (calories) into energy, the process that breaks down food to energize cells and build important cellular components. Some people are born with faster metabolism—they just naturally burn more calories. As you get older your metabolic rate slows down and more calories are stored in your body as fat. But your daily habits can raise your metabolism.

Daily Habits

These are simple things you can do right now that can have a huge impact on your health and weight.

Have a big glass of water when you wake up in the morning. Drinking eight to twelve ounces of room-temperature water first thing in the morning before anything else. This flushes out the toxins and is the perfect way to start the day.

I talked in chapter 2 about the effects of water and dehydration on your skin for beauty, but proper hydration is also essential for your overall health. Drinking more water doesn't involve cutting back on calories or dragging yourself to the gym. It is the easiest and most profound step to losing weight and feeling better. So why are you not doing it? Most of our health problems are the result of dehydration. Most people are dehydrated because they don't eat enough fruits and vegetables, which are water dense, compounded with the fact that we drink too much coffee and alcohol, which are diuretics, meaning they force water out of the body. To compensate, the body retains water in the form of bloating.

Dehydration is also one of the biggest causes of fatigue. So if you are low on energy, chances are you should be drinking more water. If you feel thirsty, that means you are already dehydrated.

This may sound crazy, but many people lose their sense of thirst and mistake it for hunger. Often our brains say we're hungry when our bodies are actually thirsty. When you feel that urge to snack, have a tall glass of water first. Chances are that it will curb your urge. It's best to drink a full glass of water before each meal anyway; this fills your belly so you eat less.

There is no downside to drinking more water. It's easy to do and you will notice results immediately!

Soda be gone. Drinking your calories can be worse than eating them. Your body doesn't always register the calories you drink, so you don't get full as fast as after you had something to eat. Drinking just one glass of soda a day causes a woman to gain weight. The sugar in the sodas is converted right into fat, and the carbonation depletes calcium. Hot Moms, please don't get your kids started on soda; they will only crave it as an adult. Consider soda like a dessert, a treat. Cutting it out of your diet and substituting pure water, not flavored water or sports drinks, can help you drop weight and feel more energized very quickly. This includes diet soda and low-calorie soda, which are loaded with artificial sweeteners, and soda isn't hydrating or filling, so you will likely eat something else. Most people who drink soda do so in place of water. For the next three months, try cutting back and adding a glass of water instead and see what a difference it makes.

If you crave a little carbonation, mix Perrier or seltzer water with pomegranate juice for a natural soda taste that is high in antioxidants. There are also several natural sodas on the market.

✿ **Hansen's** sodas don't have any caffeine, sodium, preservatives, or artificial colors. They come in ginger ale, tangerine, raspberry, vanilla cola, kiwi strawberry, and other flavors (Hansens.com).

✿ **Izze** carbonated drinks are 70 percent fruit juice and come in peach, blackberry, blueberry, and other flavors (Izze.com).

✿ **Oogavé** sodas are sweetened only with organic agave nectar. Among their flavors are natural root beer, mandarin key lime, and watermelon (Oogave.com).

Eat breakfast. "Breakfast" literally means "breaking a fast." Your metabolic rate drops overnight because of fasting. So if you miss your morning meal and then eat a hearty lunch, the majority of calories are stored as fat because your metabolism can't handle the sudden load. You may also become so hungry by lunchtime that you might eat more and might not make the healthiest decisions about what you eat. Eating a healthy breakfast will get your metabolism started and kick-start your day with an energy boost. Breakfast for kids is especially important; children who eat breakfast have better concentration and are more alert and creative.

Desperately seeking sugar? The average American eats twenty tablespoons of sugar each day in the form of processed foods such as soda, baked goods, fast cereals, fruit drinks, and flavored yogurt. All that sugar increases insulin production, which rushes to store the sugar (as fat) and usually leads a dramatic drop in blood sugar—so an hour or two later, you're back to craving sugary foods again. So toss the junk food. Clean out your cabinets and restock with healthy options. You won't be tempted by junk food if it isn't there, and eventually you won't even desire those foods. Your body will recognize how bad it makes you feel. Cravings are all about blood sugar. If your levels stay consistent throughout the day, your eating patterns (and moods) will, too. Your blood sugar can fall after four hours of not eating—so snack! Most processed foods contain sweeteners, many of which are artificial sugar substitutes containing no natural sugars, such as saccharine and aspartame. Check your labels. A diet high in additives and preservatives can cause hyperactivity and aggression. Chromium is removed from foods in the refining process, and chromium is needed to control blood sugar levels. Artificial sweeteners are also linked to behavioral problems and allergies. It's simple: If you eat dead, lifeless food, you will be lifeless; if you eat vital, vibrant foods such as fresh fruits and veggies, you will be full of vitality, too.

A great resource that is straightforward and easy to read is the bestseller *You Are What You Eat: The Plan That Will Change Your Life*, by Dr. Gillian McKeith.

HERE ARE SOME OF MY FAVORITE HEALTHY SNACK OPTIONS.

❂ Clif nutrition bars (ClifBar.com)

❂ Food Should Taste Good chips (Food ShouldTasteGood.com)

- Frozen grapes

- Kashi products (Kashi.com)

- Luna nutrition bars (LunaBar.com)

- Nuts—pour on some honey and roast with cinnamon for a go-to snack. (That saying "soup to nuts" originated because nuts were often served as an after-dinner treat.)

- Plain yogurt with sesame, pumpkin, and sunflower seeds on top, sweetened with agave nectar or honey

- Popcorn, unsweetened and unbuttered

- Sliced apple and natural peanut butter dip

- Somersaults (SomersaultSnackCo.com)

- Terra exotic vegetable chips

- Trail mix

- Veggies dipped in hummus or guacamole

MAKE THE SWITCH. THESE SIMPLE SWAPS IN FOOD CHOICES CAN EASILY LEAD TO A MORE HEALTHY BODY AND MIND.

- Use wheat bread and buns instead of white bread.

- Try sweet-potato fries rather than french fries.

- Serve wheat or whole-grain pasta, not regular pasta.

- Change white rice for quinoa or brown rice.

- Choose turkey over beef.

- Substitute honey or agave nectar for sugar.

- Use pure maple syrup instead of the high-fructose corn syrup kind you are likely using now. At first it might taste funny, but you will get used to it, I promise. Now I can't even eat the other kind because it tastes way to sweet for me. If you start your kids with pure maple, they won't know the difference.

- Lose processed peanut butter and buy the real thing instead. Look at the label. It should say *peanuts and salt*—no other ingredients!

- Olive oil is better for you than vegetable oil.

- Eat an apple rather than drinking apple juice. Juice has 120 calories and no fiber. Apples have 80 calories and three to four grams of fiber each.

❀ Choose vinaigrette dressing over ranch or
   blue cheese.

❀ Instead of sports drinks, drink coconut
   water. It is a better and more natural source
   of electrolytes.

❀ Ditch milk chocolate in favor of dark choco-
   late. It is actually good for you it has twice
   as many flavonoids as sweet milk chocolate.
   You can order great indulgent treats from
   TheProteinBakery.com and Coracao
   Confections.com.

Whole Foods

Eat more whole foods—foods that are still in their
natural state, such as fruits, vegetables, brown rice, raw
nuts, honey. Skip processed foods—foods that are made
from whole foods but have been refined and infused
with chemical preservatives, such as hot dogs, french
fries, canned fruits, chicken nuggets, and bacon bits.
Avoid junk foods, like doughnuts, chips, cheese puffs,
etc., and foods that are white, for example, pasta, white
rice, potatoes, and white bread.

What's Cookin'?

It is not as hard or as bland as you think to add
healthy options to your daily meals. Here are some fun
recipes for everyday food you already eat, just made a

little more nutritious. I made and served all of these last Saturday. I hope you enjoy them as much as my family did.

Note that I don't use standard measuring in any of my recipes. I like to get creative, have fun, see what it needs, and either add a little or subtract depending on taste.

BREAKFAST

Bananas about French Toast

I am sure you all know how to make french toast: create your batter, dip or soak the bread, then place in a frying pan. I usually make this on the weekend, and I make extra so I can freeze it for breakfast on busy school days.

> 3 eggs or egg whites
> Almond milk
> Vanilla extract
> Cinnamon
> 1 mushy banana
> Sliced whole wheat bread

Blend all ingredients except the bread together in a wide bowl, then dip or soak the bread. Fry in a lightly oiled frying pan until lightly browned.

Serve with real maple syrup. Slice into french toast strips and let your kids dip them in the syrup. This is a wonderful breakfast for you and your kids.

Backyard Gourmet Turkey Burger

> Lean ground turkey
> Finely chopped onions
> A spoonful of ground flaxseed
> Minced parsley
> 2 egg whites

Mix all ingredients together, roll into patties, and then grill. Serve on toasted whole wheat buns. Add tomato, lettuce, and avocado as toppings, and *yum—* healthy and delicious.

For kids, you could take out the onions and parsley and serve with melted jack and cheddar cheeses.

Salmon Burgers

Combine baked wild salmon with chopped celery, green onion, a pinch of dill, a spoonful of mayo, and one egg. Mash into patties, then grill, add a squeeze of lemon, and serve with lettuce and tomato on a whole wheat bun.

DINNER

Power Quesadillas

> Black beans
> Baked and sliced sweet potatoes, yams, or butternut
>   squash

Whole wheat tortillas
Cheddar cheese
Cilantro

Mix black beans and sliced sweet potatoes, yams, or squash, then spread on a tortilla. Sprinkle with shredded cheddar cheese and cilantro. Fold and brown in the oven or on the stovetop in a skillet, cut, and serve with Greek strained yogurt instead of sour cream.

As a side dish I add sliced avocado spritzed with lime, a pinch of sea salt, and pepper.

DESSERT

Watermelon-Banana Sorbet

2 bananas, peeled and sliced
Watermelon cubes
Orange juice
Lime juice

Spread the banana slices and watermelon cubes in a single layer in a shallow metal dish. Pour orange and lime juice lightly over them then freeze for about four to five hours. Remove, let thaw partially, then break into pieces and blend in your blender until creamy. Put into cups or paper cones and serve. Yum!

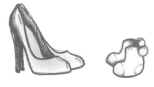

Fiber

You always hear you should eat more fiber. Well, here is why it works: simple carbohydrates are easy to digest and don't challenge the digestive system. Fiber increases your metabolism because of the additional work the body has to do to digest it. Energy is released more slowly and continually during the digestion of high-fiber foods, keeping your blood sugar level more consistent, and when your blood sugar level is consistent then you tend to snack less. Fiber also causes you to drink lots of water.

Introduce more fiber into your diet slowly. Too much too soon can cause bloating, cramps, and gas.

THESE FOODS ARE GOOD SOURCES OF FIBER.

❀ Apples

❀ Artichokes

❀ Beans

❀ Bran

❀ Broccoli

❀ Brown rice

❀ Chickpeas

- ✿ Figs
- ✿ Hummus
- ✿ Lentils
- ✿ Pears
- ✿ Peas
- ✿ Pecans
- ✿ Pistachios
- ✿ Popcorn (air popped)
- ✿ Raisins
- ✿ Raspberries
- ✿ Whole wheat products
- ✿ Yams (with the skin)

Superfoods

Here are a few of my favorite nutritional power-houses that will help you feel fantastic. Start incorporating these foods into your daily recipes.

Beans are a virtual wonder food. Long regarded as the "poor man's meat" because it is such a good source of protein, beans lost favor for a while. A study was done showing that as income level rises, bean consumption tends to decrease.

Beans play a big part in weight management. They fill you up, giving you bulk without calories, and the high fiber content controls your blood sugar, so it keeps your hunger in check while maintaining your energy levels.

HERE ARE SOME EASY AND APPETIZING WAYS TO ADD BEANS TO YOUR MEALS.

- ✿ Kidney beans are a yummy addition to any salad.

- ✿ Cannellini beans are wonderful mixed with whole wheat pasta and sauce.

- ✿ Black beans are obviously a standard ingredient in burritos, but you can also add black beans to your scrambled eggs in the morning; if you want, wrap it in a whole wheat tortilla to create a breakfast power burrito.

- ✿ Hummus is ground chickpeas with some spices. You can make your own or buy it ready made. (Sabra actually has individual snack packs, perfect for lunch boxes.) For a more appetizing color and flavor, add beets to your hummus blend. Hummus also makes a great spread on sandwiches and burgers.

A note about canned beans: they are usually high in sodium, but straining off their liquid and rinsing them with cool water eliminates up to 40 percent of the salt.

If you are worried about gas from eating beans, try Beano. It is an enzyme product that helps reduce the gas associated with foods like beans. (Hint: Many celebrities use Beano before award shows.)

BROCCOLI

Broccoli is one of the most nutrient-dense foods there is, and all that nutrition comes with very low calories. Broccoli is said to help prevent many cancers. Freeze broccoli and keep it on hand to toss in stir fries and blend in soup. I shred and sprinkle broccoli on vegetable pizzas and on omelets.

SPINACH

Not all leafy greens are created equal. The darker the greens, the better they are for you and the more powerful they are in fighting cancer and other diseases. Spinach is especially rich in calcium and has more health benefits than almost any other food. Popeye was right—eat your spinach!

Mix a spinach in salads, layer it in lasagna, chop it into an omelet, or shred it into tacos and burritos instead of lettuce.

Or make a spinach pesto: Puree raw spinach with almonds or walnuts, some garlic, olive oil, and Parmesan cheese. Serve with chickpeas or on bowtie pasta, or use as a sandwich spread.

BERRIES

Blueberries, raspberries, and all other berries are enormously high in antioxidants. Antioxidants remove free radicals, which are by-products of the oxidation process that can damage cells in your skin and other organs. Feel good and look good!

WILD SALMON

Dr. Perricone helped spark a salmon craze with his claims that it prevents wrinkles. Whether it does or not, salmon is one of the richest sources of marine-derived omega-3 fatty acids. Omega-3 fatty acids are essential to our health, but our bodies can't produce them; they must be obtained through food such as salmon, tuna, halibut, whole grains, fruits, olive oil, and garlic.

TEA TIME

Tea is one of the world's most popular superfoods. It's calming and delicious. I love the smell of tea, and just holding a big, warm mug makes me feel happy and at ease. There are many feel-good reasons to love tea. Green tea is the most famous variety at the moment and gets the most attention, but most teas are beneficial. Tea helps boost your immune system, and it protects against cancers, cavities, and sun damage, among many other benefits. So indulge yourself daily in tea time. A squeeze of lemon and a squirt of honey or agave nectar is a wonderful complement to most teas.

Tazo is one of my favorite brands of tea. They offer a

variety of interesting and delicious flavors (Tazo.com).

Matcha Matcha is micro-ground tea powder you can add to cold or hot water (MatchaMonk.com). It is an outstanding product and is perfect if you do not enjoy traditional tea. It is much sweeter and is said to have eight times the antioxidants of steeped green tea. I drink several cups a day.

Soul Food

Sometimes it is important to feed your soul. Balance is always best. I always try to eat clean, but this past summer I spent ten days in Italy around the Amalfi Coast and indulged in pizza, homemade pasta, and gelato without reservation or worry. Sometimes you just have to live and enjoy. Try to shape up your daily diet, and if you generally eat healthy, having a treat and indulging in some of your favorites is fine. So go ahead, have a scoop or two of your favorite ice cream, or steal a bite of that molten chocolate cake.

> *Soul food is just what the name implies. It is soulfully cooked food or richly flavored food, good for your ever-loving soul.*
> —Sheila Ferguson

Sol Food in San Rafael, California, serves authentic Cuban food. If you are ever in the area, I highly recommend. It is outstanding and well worth a visit (Sol FoodRestaurant.com).

Stay Healthy

Nothing derails a fitness plan faster than illness. And as moms we can't afford to get sick. Starting and keeping a healthy lifestyle will help you ward off colds and flus. Help keep your immune system at its strongest by getting enough vitamin C. An eight-ounce glass of grapefruit juice contains at least 100 percent of the recommended daily value for vitamin C—and is a perfect way to start your day.

> *I'm just one stomach flu away from my goal weight.*
> —Emily Blunt in
> *The Devil Wears Prada*

Illness and disease form in acidic environments, and it has been said that cancer and ailments cannot survive in the opposite, an alkaline environment. And it is estimated that a third of cancers could be prevented by a change in diet. Eat foods that keep your body alkaline, like parsley, asparagus, red peppers, watermelon, lemons, mushrooms, cucumber, carrots, cauliflower, spinach, sweet potatoes, tomatoes, peas, onions, garlic, eggplant, beets, broccoli, papaya, pineapple, apples, avocados, blackberries, oranges, pears, raisins, coconut, grapes, almonds, and tofu. Meat is very acidic, as are beer, white sugar, soda, breads, and pastries. You might think that citrus fruits are acidic because of the citric acid they contain, but they actually have an alkalinizing effect in your body.

Greens+ Energy Bars (GreensPlus.com) are alkaline forming, taste good, and are packed with superfoods.

Negative attitudes also contribute to disease. Disease is just that; your body and mind are connected, and your body responds to your mind's beliefs. So go easier on yourself; be more loving in your thoughts and how you feed and treat your body.

The Scoop on Your Poop

You are always hearing exaggerated stories about the latest celebrity cleanse or detox. Gwyneth Paltrow dedicated a whole newsletter on her blog, Goop.com, to a cleanse she took part in. And Ben Affleck described his colonic experience on a late night talk show. Our bodies are naturally detoxing every day through urine, bowel movements, and sweat. But because of modern environmental toxins and processed foods, our bodies can become overloaded, making it more important to drink water to flush out toxins continuously.

Your poop is an important indicator of your overall health. Food should take twelve to twenty-four hours to digest. If you want to check to see how fast your system is working, here are a few ways. Eat sweet corn or whole sunflower seeds; both are recognizable in your stool. Another way is to eat beets; they will turn your stool bright red. Watch to see how long it takes these foods to turn up. Not to get too personal, but you should be pooping at least once a day, and it should be golden brown and shaped like an unripe banana. It should come out easily and be odorless. If you are constipated, you are already dehydrated, so add water and fiber to your diet, and ask your doctor what cleanse would be right for you. A clean colon is essential to good health.

Weight a Minute

HERE ARE SOME TIPS AND TRICKS FOR KEEPING THE POUNDS OFF.

✿ Eat soup. You will tend to eat less after a hot bowl of soup. Plus, because it's hot, you usually eat it slowly.

✿ Eat late, eat light. Finish eating two hours before bedtime and you will sleep much better. It is ironic that we eat more during dinner than any other time of the day; we don't need extra energy when we sleep.

✿ Take advantage of your faster metabolism by eating within an hour after exercising. You burn calories quicker and more efficiently after a workout. Plus, your muscles need the nutrients for repair.

✿ Journal your food intake—and be honest! When you have to write down what food you eat, you tend to eat less and make healthier food choices. And you might be less tempted by the free food at the bake sale or donuts in the office.

✿ Graze. Eat small meals or snacks throughout the day. Not eating for three or four hours can put your body in starvation mode, when it starts conserving calories instead of burning them. Eating small amounts continuously also prevents you from bingeing.

❁ Eat slowly. Savor and enjoy your meal; really taste your food. It takes twenty minutes for your body to register that it is full.

❁ Drink with your dominant hand at parties. If you have a drink in your dominant hand while you're circulating at a party, you will be less likely to grab food and eat.

❁ Keep a positive attitude. You have to be positive, set goals, visualize achieving them, and believe that you can be a fit Hot Mom.

❁ Laughter boosts metabolism—so laugh! A lot!

Be in Your Body

Respect your body; be kind to it and treat it well. Eat for nourishment. Exercise for energy and peace of mind. Visualize good health and your ideal weight. This chapter is the foundation of a healthy, more energetic lifestyle. Do your research, consult your physician, and see a nutritionist to find out the optimal plan for your body type and goals. There is no doubt you are well on your way to becoming a fit Hot Mom!

If you want to see what your body will look like tomorrow, look at your thoughts today.
—Hindu saying

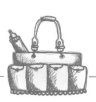
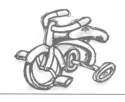

Six

Better Homes and Guardrails
(After All, Doesn't the Average Childproof Home Resemble a Maximum Security Prison?)

My second favorite household chore is ironing. My first being hitting my head on the top bunk bed until I faint.

—Erma Bombeck

Eminent Domain

The personality of your home reflects who you are, where you've been, what's going on in your life. You will express yourself in your house whether you intend to or not.

When friends enter a home, they sense its personality and character, the family's style of living—these elements make a house come alive with a sense of identity, a sense of energy, enthusiasm, and warmth, declaring, "This is who we are; this is how we live."

—Ralph Lauren

The Mood

Your home should be inviting, fun, and have a sense of balance. A house with a positive mood and vibe will help keep its occupants in a happy mood. No matter what your style, it should feel like home to you and to your kids. Imagine coming home on cold winter day; the kids are drinking hot chocolate with extra marshmallows, and you are all curling up by a warm fire with a snuggly throw and a sleepy dog by your feet. That warm, safe feeling is what home is all about, no matter what the season.

BRING THE OUTSIDE IN.

✿ Open up some windows and let the fresh air inside. Airing out your home's most commonly used rooms for an hour or two a day keeps musty smells at bay and serves as a lovely reminder that spring has arrived. (Of course, be cautious if you have little ones.)

✿ Get back to nature. Home décor plucked from nature adds a beautiful touch. Look for elements of nature when you are out on walks with the kids—shells, stones, interesting pieces of natural wood. Cluster them together to create impact with virtually no upkeep.

✿ Pair blooming plants with brightly colored pots to perk things up.

❀ Add sparkle. Natural crystals and quartz make beautiful décor.

❀ Painted birdcages can be fun, too. Fill them with candles or flowers.

❀ Look at your front door. What does it say about your home? A small spring wreath or charm on the doorknob can personalize your entry and be a happy greeting for guests—and for you when you come home.

> —San Francisco interior designer
> Jordan Adair Stephens, Hot Mom of two

EMBRACE COLOR.

❀ Think of color as an accessory. Paint is a foolproof way to make your home design come together. It's easy and inexpensive to change.

❀ Add a bounty of colorful pillows to celebrate the season. To offset the cheerful pillows, use blankets and throws in dark neutrals. A nicely folded throw will not only make a room seem put together, it can also be used last minute to protect furniture when kids come running.

❀ Instead of having framed photos randomly placed throughout the house, bring them all together in one space for impact. Hallways and entryways are often overlooked, but they shouldn't be. We walk through these areas all the time, making them the perfect location for a collage of family photos.

❀ In the kitchen, frame chalkboards in fun or detailed frames. It adds elegance and is a great way to write notes to the family and keep schedules.

❀ Be your own decorator. There are many helpful decorating shows on the cable networks with before-and-after reveals and ideas from top design experts. HGTV.com and DIYnetwork.com are two great resources to find decorating tips and tricks on any budget.

Makes Scents

The sense of smell has the power to recall memories. Your home is where your kids are going to develop many of the associations they bring to adulthood, from the scents that come from your dryer sheets, the food cooking, or candles burning.

Sleep with the kids' bedspreads or pillowcases one night so they smell like you. When my son was a baby someone told me to sleep with his crib sheets before I put them on so they would have mom's comforting smell. I did. My son was always a good sleeper; I don't know if that is the reason, but why not give it a try? It doesn't matter what age your "baby" is, a parent's scent will always make them feel comforted. It is also a good idea to give them your pillowcase to sleep with when you are out of town.

It's our job as moms to create a home that smells pleasing—smells spur memories—so indulge yourself with comforting aromas that remind you of your childhood.

Flower Power

Fresh flowers can bring uplifting energy to your home. They are therapeutic and just make you feel good. Giving and receiving flowers has a certain charm. I always have sunflowers in a vase in my kitchen or living room. It's my Sunday tradition to pick them with my son at the local farmers' market.

I'd rather have fresh flowers on my table than diamonds around my neck.
—Emma Goldman

HERE ARE SOME TRICKS TO MAKE FLOWERS LOOK PRETTY AND LAST LONGER.

❀ Cut stems on forty-five-degree angle, and cut them underwater (with kitchen scissors in the sink) to prevent air from getting into the veins of the stem.

❀ Keep flowers in deep water for a few hours before transferring them to a vase with shallow water.

- ❀ Change the water in the vase every other day.

- ❀ Add a teaspoon of sugar to the water to refresh the flowers. A crushed aspirin also works, but let it dissolve in the water before you put the flowers in.

- ❀ Use a plastic straw to stabilize droopy stems or to make flowers fit better in long vases.

- ❀ Remove dying flowers right away. Dying flowers emit ethylene gas, which will cause the other flowers to wilt also.

- ❀ For some reason, tulips last twice as long if you put a few pennies into their water.

- ❀ A spritz of hairspray can preserve cut flowers. Hold the can a foot or so away and give a quick spray to the undersides of the petals.

- ❀ Don't place flowers near your fruit bowl. Ripe fruits also emit ethylene, which will cause your flowers to wilt and decay.

- ❀ If you are picking flowers yourself, do so first thing in the morning or in the evening; that's when the sugar reserves in the stems are at their highest. Never pick when the sun is at its hottest, because the heat of the sun lowers the water content in the flowers and they will not last as long.

❀ Flowers should be picked when they are in bud or half open so you can enjoy watching them open slowly.

❀ Picking flowers is a great activity to do with your kids. Let them make or decorate vases to fill, and then they can take care of their own flowers.

❀ When the kids are small, start a tradition of letting your child pick flowers from your yard to bring to his or her teacher on the first day of school. It is a sweet gesture, not to mention a great way to start off on the right foot!

❀ During the holidays, fill glass vases with cranberries and water then arrange white roses in them. It looks dramatic and instantly adds an upscale feel to any dinner or party.

Feng Shui

The art of feng shui (pronounced "fung shwee"), which literally means "wind water," has been practiced by the Chinese for thousands of years. It is the system of arranging your surroundings so that you can live in harmony with them. According to the principles of feng shui, every aspect of your life is anchored energetically in your living space, so clearing your clutter can completely transform your existence. It is believed that feng shui can be used to predict and alter situations such as health, wealth, family life, and relationships.

According to the "Feng Shui Guy," Ariel Joseph Towne, any kind of clutter in a home creates an obstacle to the smooth flow of energy around a space. This in turn creates stuckness and confusion in the lives of the home's occupants.

> **Clutter: (n) A confused multitude of things.**
>
> *The word "clutter" comes from the Middle English word **clotteren**, which means "to clot."*

Clutter and chaos can affect the way our minds work. They can also affect how we feel and interfere with our ability to relax and get the rest we need to rejuvenate. Keeping things as organized as possible will add to an environment that creates a feeling of peace and comfort that will affect the entire family. It is important to note that this principle applies not just to your possessions; anything left unfinished is a form of clutter, like projects or errands. Mental and emotional situations as well as physical surroundings can clutter your psyche. So limit what you have to do and finish what you start.

HERE ARE ARIEL JOSEPH TOWNE'S TIPS FOR USING FENG SHUI IN YOUR NURSERY OR CHILD'S ROOM.

✿ **Keep the bed protected.** In feng shui, you always want to make sure that the places where you spend the most time in a room (beds, desks, couches) are placed into command positions. This means against

a solid wall, on the far side of the room out
of the path of the door. For children, this
can mean in a corner where two solid walls
meet.

✿ **Beware of invisible enemies: energy
stealers.** Don't place the bed directly
under a window, an air conditioner, or a fan.
They not only can create a draft, but they
also are thought to disrupt the energy of
those who sleep underneath them.

✿ **Don't point mirrors at the bed.** Mirrors are great for rooms because they create
depth and can sometimes reflect natural
light, thereby brightening up a room. Unfortunately, they can also create too much
energy in a room, which can affect adults'
sleep. Since children are more sensitive than
we are, their beds should be kept out of the
path of a mirror. If the mirror and bed are
immovable, then the mirrors should be covered at night and used only during awake
time. If your child continues to have restless
sleep, remove the mirrors from the room
altogether and see if that helps.

✿ **Don't use metal bed frames.** For some
reason, metal bed frames tend to conduct
a low-level current of energy, which can
disrupt sleep. It's definitely better to have a
wooden bed frame rather than a metal one,
preferably one with round edges.

❁ **Stay away from sharp corners.** Not only can sharp edges on furniture hurt you if you bump into them, but people have noticed that over time, sitting or sleeping near sharp-edged items can affect our health and well-being.

❁ **Keep away from stimulating colors.** Some colors are good for being active, and other colors are more beneficial to rest. Studies at the University of British Columbia have shown that color can affect our moods. Children have been known to get more agitated or colicky when placed into rooms with bright colors, especially when they are trying to rest. Stay away from bright oranges, reds, and pinks. See if you can bring in colors that seem peaceful and restful. Pastels in the blue, green, or soft yellow are always a safe bet. If you want pink, try a light rose. When picking a color, ask yourself what mood it gives you and then realize that to a child it might be amplified.

❁ **Consider adding live plants.** In addition to helping add some life to the room, some plants can also help to purify the air. But avoid plants with sharp leaves for the same reasons you should avoid sharp-edged furniture.

✿ **Surround your child with loving and peaceful images.** Make sure that artwork doesn't appear scary, either in the daytime or at night in case your child wakes up and sees it in the dark. The same goes for toys and dolls. If possible, place a mobile above the bed, or decorate the walls with photographs of you with your kids, or other items that will make them feel loved, protected, and peaceful.

✿ **Create a clean slate.** As you are welcoming new life into your home, you want to make sure that you aren't loading your space up with baggage from whatever happened before. For every layer of paint that is on the wall, there is also a layer of energy from whatever happened there before. Whether it is emotional (fighting, sadness, or worry) or somber (someone died in the room), you can create a clean slate by doing a cleansing ritual in your home. Some people like to use a bell to shake clean the walls of the old energy. Other people like to burn a candle or two. Place your hands together and say to yourself a few words that feel good to you. After you feel that the space is clean, then start to visualize peace, happiness, and health for your child. Your space is now ready to receive on all levels.

❀ Children's clutter seems to breed and take over, so it is especially important to keep it under control. Allow clutter to collect on the outside and your child will tend to collect clutter on the inside, too.

For more feng shui tips and tricks, or to schedule a consultation with Anel, visit TheFengShuiGuy.com.

ECO-MINDED MAMA

Junk your junk mail. Almost four million tons of junk mail is sent in the United States each year, half of which is never opened. A hundred million trees are destroyed each year to produce junk mail. Twenty-eight billion gallons of water are wasted each year to produce or recycle junk mail. And if helping the environment isn't enough motivation, do it for yourself. Each person spends an average of seventy hours a year dealing with and sorting through junk mail. Sign up with 41pounds.org, a service that calls companies and gets you off mailing lists. They can stop 80 to 95 percent of unwanted catalogues and junk mail. The name comes from the fact that each American receives approximately forty-one pounds of junk mail a year. The cost for the service is $41 for five years, a third of which is donated to an environmental group of your choice.

If you don't want to use a service to stop your mail, call the toll-free numbers on the back of the unwanted catalogues and remove yourself from the lists. Also, most companies and organizations, unless they state otherwise, sell the information you give whenever you fill out a warranty, donate to a charity, or order a product or service. To avoid being put on more and more mailing lists, make sure you write in big letters, "Please do not sell my name or address." Most organizations will record this preference in their databases and honor your request. To track which groups are selling your address, put a false middle name or initial when you fill out new forms; when you get unwanted mail with the "mistakes" you created, you will know who sold or shared your information.

Little Things, Big Difference

Make Your Bed Every Morning

My mom is not going to believe I wrote this. For years she begged and pleaded and bribed me to make my bed. Making your bed is quick and easy to do, and it makes everything look so much neater. Outer order contributes to inner calm. Sticking to a resolution no matter how small can bring satisfaction, and it allows you to start the day feeling accomplished and disciplined. Because making your bed is such a small task, it is a great resolution to start and stick with.

Lose the Shoes

Take your shoes off when you enter the house. In many cultures it is customary for spiritual or practical reasons to remove your shoes before entering. But it can also keep your home much cleaner. Think about all of the things the bottoms of your shoes come in contact with: restroom floors, gas from the gas station, chemical fertilizer from grass—these get tracked through your house. Now think about how much time your kids spend playing or crawling on the floor exposed to those same contaminants. The contaminants can also become airborne, so you might inhale them as well. There is a simple solution: Put a cute shoe bin or rug inside each entrance to your home. Instruct your kids and guests to take off shoes when they enter. Guests will get the hint when they see your shoe pile. In case they feel uncomfortable because their pedicure is out of date or for other reasons, have a fresh pack of socks to offer. And get slippers or special "house shoes" that don't go outside for yourself and the kids so that they feel more excited about doing this. Before you know it, it will become just one more of your many good habits.

Thank You

These two words, thank you, can have quite an emotional impact. It seems so simple, but taking a minute to write a quick thank-you is a great way to improve and preserve relationships.

You have 86,400 seconds today. Have you used one to say thank you?
—William Arthur Ward

It's not always practical, but when I have birthday parties or events I try to take photos of everyone who comes and send a note with their photo as a thank-you for their gift or for attending. It's a big hit!

Letting kids choose their own personalized stationery and thank-you cards will make it easier to get them to write them. Have a special pen, stickers, and stamps as well so that writing their thank-you notes feels special and fun for them. You can also get personalized preprinted return-address labels with characters or designs they like. Get kids in the habit early on and it will become automatic for them. Growing up I can remember that my mom didn't let us enjoy our gift until we wrote our thank-you note for it. Here are some sites that allow you to customize your thank-you cards: TinyPrints.com, PaperStyle.com, InvitationBox.com, MyExpression.com, Shutterfly.com. Shutterfly even allows you to print photos on the thank-you cards—too cute!

Have Go-To Gifts Handy

You never want to be caught without a gift, running around last minute trying to pull a gift together, because your seven-year-old just informed you that his best friend's birthday party is in an hour. In my hall closet I have a box of gifts for last-minute parties or invitations. Unisex gifts are always great: picture frames and candles work. And if the box is special enough you don't even need to wrap it. When classic toys go on sale, be sure to stock up: items like Play-Doh, bubbles, balls, books, stuffed animals, and card games such as Uno will work for both boys and girls. Gift bags and tissue paper are perfect for wrapping on the fly, so always have some handy.

Now, if you really want to make an impression, use

that frame from your supply of last-minute gifts and frame a card or piece of paper that says (in your handwriting), "Let's create a memory and put the photo in here." You can be specific if you have been planning to go somewhere—maybe a new restaurant—with that person. It's the surprise that cements the memory. I recently gave a friend two funny teacups and a packet of tea with a little note that said, "I miss you. Let's do tea time soon." She loved it. If you are a feeling a little cheeky, when you give your man clothes of any kind attach a note that says, "I can't wait to tear this off of you." Just that little note can really spice up practical gifts. Be clever and express your feelings—that sentiment is the real gift.

File It Up

The whole reason for getting organized is to relieve stress by bringing things under control. It is one thing to have your drawers neatly in order but it doesn't compare to having your paperwork and medical records handy should you need them fast. Creating an efficient system for filing your important documents and paperwork is one of the most important things you can do in your home, it is not as daunting a task as you might think. Purchase a safe to put original copies of your kids' birth certificates and social security cards, but also make photo copies you can keep in a file with their name on it for handy reference. If you registered your child's cord blood, keep that information, as well as their medical records, in the file as well. Don't forget to tell all of your doctors that you have the cord blood, with advancements in technology the stem cells can be used to treat so many injuries. For more information, go to CordBlood.com. The Baby Briefcase is perfect to place all of your copies of important documents (OrganizedFromTheStart.com).

Cell-Phone-Free Times

Create cell-phone-free times with the kids—and stick to it. Admittedly I was one of those people who need to check their BlackBerrys every few seconds, and I would lunge at every beep. I thought I was good about limiting calls when I was with my son. But then he had a class assignment that was a big wake-up call for me (pun intended). My son had to draw his family and write things about them—and he innocently drew a picture of me talking on a cell phone. Was this how he perceived me? It really hit me hard and made me realize how much time I used my phone when I was with him.

DID YOU KNOW?

A recent survey on cell phone use produced these surprising results:

- ✿ 22 percent of people surveyed said they have stopped sex to answer the phone.

- ✿ 77 percent admitted to texting while driving.

- ✿ 79 percent have texted while going to the bathroom.

❁ 18 percent have texted during a wedding.

❁ 37 percent have texted during a graduation.

❁ 16 percent have texted during a funeral.

❁ 26 percent said they have been broken up
with or have broken up with someone via a
text message.

❁ There are approximately 18.5 billion texts
sent each month.

On a more serious note, I have seen many moms in the carpool chatting on their phones or texting while they're behind the wheel, and not too long ago I was one of them. Almost a half million people are injured every year because of accidents involving texting and driving, and more than six thousand people (including children) are killed. Oprah Winfrey's No Phone Zone is a pledge not to use your phone while driving. My car has Bluetooth and I love it. It is a completely hands-free way to talk on the phone, and it's well worth installing. You are carrying the most precious cargo when you drive; endangering your children's lives is not worth that phone call or text. It can wait a few minutes until you get home. Oprah has declared April 30 No Phone Zone Day, and on Oprah.com there are many heartbreaking stories of people whose lives have been affected by distracted drivers. If you need any more convincing, just read a few of them.

While I'm writing this, my housekeeper is sweeping up the Olympic-sized pile of trash our family has generated since she last visited us.

In my mind, this makes me only one step removed from the tanned people driving black Beemers with tinted windows who cut you off in traffic without a backward glance, or the heavily Botoxed trophy wives who spend their lives chewing out salesgirls at Nordstrom.

In the past, this feeling would make me flee the house when my cleaning lady arrived. Nowadays, though, since I mostly work at home, I can't always get away during her visits. So I'm forced to confront the reality of someone else cleaning up my stuff.

Hiring a company has actually crossed my mind, except that I like knowing the money I pay my cleaning lady goes directly into her pocket, and not to some business owner with overhead and profit margins.

I also pay her a bit more than the going rate, based on the fact that she works hard and she's doing work I hate doing myself.

That's the guilt talking, of course, but I'd rather pay a bit too much than have the attitude of some people I know: How cheap can I get her? Sorry, I'm not interested in exploiting other people's desperation any more than I already do. I shop at Walmart, so I figure I already have done my part exploiting people in Third World countries.

And, now, it's time for lunch. My housekeeper has just finished doing the kitchen, so I'm not afraid to walk in there anymore.

And, it will stay clean and sweet-smelling for least for a couple of hours, until the kids get home. By dark, of course, it will look like she was never here at all.

—Marla Jo Fisher, from "Watching Someone Clean Your House: Awkward," in the *Orange County Register*

I'm not going to vacuum
'til Sears makes one you can ride on.
—Roseanne Barr

Home Clean Home

I am always looking for ways to make life easier and more efficient. Nothing adds to your stress like a messy house, and nothing feels as good as when your home is clean and sparkling and looking and smelling fresh. Here are some great cleaning tips to help get the family involved.

Set your cleaning to music. Crank up your favorite tunes and dance while you clean. This will put some pep in your step and make the job seem less tedious.

Use a clean, dry paintbrush to dust wicker furniture and baskets. It also gets into those hard-to-reach corners.

Put an old pair of socks on your hands as if they were puppets, spray with a duster spray, and dust away. Kids love this. (Swiffer Dust & Shine spray is my personal favorite.)

For vacuuming made easy, a Hoover Platinum Collection Cordless Stick Vac has all the power of a plug-in—but it's cordless! It's also lightweight, so it is easy to get up and down stairs. It works on hardwood or carpets and is ideal for apartment living or for quick cleaning with a houseful of kids.

Invest in a microwave plate cover. Microwaves can be challenging to clean, so use a cover to reduce the splatter.

I like to use Dawn Hand Renewal with Olay Beauty when I do dishes because it doesn't dry out my hands.

Lemons are a secret weapon for cleaning. Lemons in a bowl or jar make a beautiful centerpiece, and when they get too ripe, cut them and put down your garbage disposal to keep it smelling fresh. You can also remove counter stains with a squeeze of lemon juice and a little baking soda.

> *Cleaning up with children around is like shoveling during a blizzard.*
> —Unknown

Mr. Clean Magic Eraser couldn't be more appropriately named. It magically erases marks from the wall. If you have boys, this is a must!

To pick up glitter, roll over it with balled-up masking tape. Or put double-stick tape on the bottom of your kids' socks and have them walk around on it to get the area clean.

It is important to keep your house neat, but remember your priorities, and be willing to let the dishes sit now and then in favor of card game with the kids or a glass of wine with your husband. You can look at your house and get overwhelmed, or you can see all the things that need to get done and tackle those jobs one by one. Staying on top of things is much easier in the long run, so make a plan of what needs to be cleaned each day, chores that can be done each week, and those that can be put off to once a month. A friend of mine with a large family told me that on Saturday mornings her mom would post a chore list on the refrigerator. The person who got up first could pick first, and the person who got up last was stuck with what was left. The kids had to initial each chore so their mom could check in with the right child when the chore was finished.

> No one ever died from sleeping in an unmade bed. I have known mothers who remake the bed after their children do it because there's a wrinkle in the spread or the blanket is on crooked. This is sick.
> —Erma Bombeck

I have asked friends and Hot Moms Club members for their best secrets and tips to making cleaning easier. Here are some of my favorites. I have tried them all, and I am glad to say they do in fact work!

HERE ARE SOME CLEANING TIPS FROM THE HOT MOMS CLUB.

✿ Removing stuck-on food in pots, pans, and Crock-Pots: Fill the pan with water and place a fabric softener sheet in the water.

Allow the pan to soak overnight. The food will wipe right out!

✿ Maintaining glitter on clothing: That new sparkly shirt shedding glitter all over the place? Spray with aerosol hair spray to make it stay put. Wash separately from other clothes, or at least wash it inside out if you must wash with other clothes.

✿ Removing wax from carpeting or fabric: First, scrape away any excess. Then, place a brown paper bag over the wax and run a warm iron over the bag. The wax will melt right into the bag! Continue moving the bag around as you pick up the wax so you are always using a clean section. If a little grease stain remains on carpet, sprinkle with baking soda and allow to sit overnight before vacuuming, which will remove the grease residue.

✿ Getting rid of microwave filth: Food splatters all over the inside of your microwave and gets cooked on after a time. To easily remove this mess, place a sponge soaked in water in the microwave. Cook on high for two minutes, then allow it to sit for five minutes without opening the microwave door. The filth is now ready to be wiped right off—no scrubbing—and your sponge is right there!

❀ Fixing sticky zippers: To make a zipper slide up and down more smoothly, rub a bar of soap over the teeth.

❀ Making dresser drawers glide: If you have a dresser drawer that is stubborn, rub a bar of soap or a candle on the top, bottom, and sides of the drawer. It will loosen right up and glide more easily.

❀ Freshening up your clothes storage: Tuck a sachet of lavender and small cedar blocks in your clothes drawers. They both smell wonderful and they also repel moths.

❀ Hanging frames: Before you hang a photo, put a piece of tape where you're putting the nail so that the plaster won't chip, crack, or flake.

❀ Finding the right key: Use nail polish to color-code your keys. It stays much better and is easier to see than marker.

❀ Brightening buttons: Paint buttons with clear nail polish to make them look shiny and new. Clear nail polish also works to stop a run in your tights.

❀ Keeping socks together: Safety-pin sock mates together before you put them in the hamper so that they don't get separated.

❀ Getting out blood stains: Rinse in cold water. Do not wash in hot water because that sets the stain. Another trick is to put a few drops of hydrogen peroxide on the blood stain with an eyedropper. If you are not at home or don't have these items handy, spit on it—yup, there is an enzyme in your saliva that breaks down the protein in blood.

❀ Getting out grass stains: Most grass stains will come out with rubbing alcohol and a soak in hot water.

❀ Getting out sweat stains: For fresh perspiration marks, pour some shampoo on the area before washing.

❀ Getting ink out: Put the clothes ink-side down on a paper towel, then blot the back of the fabric with rubbing alcohol until the stain seeps from the shirt onto the paper towel. The ink comes right out, and it can be fun to watch.

❀ Removing gum: Freeze the garment and then peel off the gum.

❀ Finding a lost earring: Don't panic if you loose a small item like an earring or a small toy part. Put pantyhose over the bottom of the vacuum hose and suck around the area where you think the item was lost. Keep checking to see if it's caught in the pantyhose.

* Cleaning jewelry: If you don't have any jewelry cleaner on hand, dish soap will also work on diamonds. I put my earrings in a little cup with dish soap and water and clean them with a toothbrush.

BABY ON A BUDGET

* Clothespins are a cheap alternative to chip bag clips.

* Let the kids decorate their own clothespins, and use these to close the chips and snacks that belong to them.

* Leftover egg cartons can be used as ice cube trays.

ECO-MINDED MAMA

* Put a brick or rock in the toilet tank (NOT the bowl) to cut down on water bill.

* If your kids waste toilet paper by rolling out too much, press the roll flat before you put it on the spindle. It will be harder to unroll because of the creases, and inevitably they will use less.

- Recycle by cutting old towels or stained clothes into cleaning rags.

- Healthy Child, Healthy World has information about eco-friendly cleaning at HealthyChild.org.

- Stay up-to-date on environmental news and eco-friendly home products at Grist.org.

Leftover Solutions

If you think that something in your fridge is too bad to eat, don't use it. If it smells bad or rancid or is the wrong color, throw it away. There are leftovers, and then there are *leftovers*.

Most times, the meals I wouldn't mind having leftovers from are the ones that vanish to the last crumb. Think of ways to get creative with the food that is left. Creative sandwiches are fun; everything seems to taste good between two pieces of bread. My mom used to call them "kitchen sink" sandwiches because we would use everything but the kitchen sink in them. Blending veggies into soups or pot pies or omelets is a fun way to use up those leftovers.

Make your own TV dinners rather than buying packaged ones. They will not only taste better and be more healthy, but assuming you have leftovers once in a while, they're basically free. Just put complete meals into a container with compartments—Tupperware and Pyrex both make them—and then freeze. Heat in the microwave when you are ready to serve. They're convenient and fun, especially on nights when you have a babysitter. The sitter can just pop out the meals when you are gone.

I like to make and freeze a big batch of pancakes so that I have them for the whole week. It's so convenient to just microwave breakfast on busy days. So next time instead of tossing that leftover batter, make up some extra pancakes and freeze them in packs of two or three—then just heat and go on busy school-day mornings.

If you brew a cup of coffee that nobody drinks, instead of throwing it away, pour it into an ice cube tray and freeze it. Coffee ice cubes are great to use when you want to make iced coffee without diluting the flavor.

Stale Bread: Not Just for the Duck Pond

Make croutons from leftover or stale bread. Cut into squares and drizzle olive oil on top; sprinkle with some salt and garlic powder to taste and bake at 300 degrees for fifteen minutes. Then let cool. Eat right away, while they're crispy.

Or use stale sliced bread to make breadcrumbs. Either toast it in the toaster or in the oven at 300 degrees for ten minutes. Let it cool, then process in the food processor until it becomes lumpy and sand-like. If you don't have a food processor, you can seal it in a plastic bag and mash until it becomes crumbs. Then place the plastic bag in the freezer until you need it for recipes.

HERE ARE SOME YUMMY WAYS TO USE BREADCRUMBS.

✿ Mix with ground turkey for meatballs.

✿ Sprinkle on top of macaroni and cheese to make it crunchy.

✿ Use to bread chicken or sliced eggplant. Beat an egg, dip chicken or eggplant in the egg, then roll in the breadcrumbs and fry or bake until golden brown. Spritz a little lemon juice on top and serve.

✿ Make stuffed mushrooms. Remove the mushroom stems and dice; mix with Parmesan, parsley, and breadcrumbs; stuff into the mushroom caps, put a dot of butter on each, and bake.

✿ Make Italian rice balls. Mix the breadcrumbs with risotto, eggs, and grated cheddar cheese. Roll into little balls, coat with more breadcrumbs, and fry in vegetable oil until golden brown. I like to serve these with marinara dipping sauce. This is a crowd pleaser!

✿ Make croquettes. Form leftover mashed potatoes into little balls, dip in beaten egg, and roll in the breadcrumbs. Then bake or fry for a delicious treat.

Zest

A pinch of citrus zest adds flavor and a hint of elegance and fun to any meal or dessert. Save the rinds of oranges and lemons in a plastic bag and freeze to use for zest. Just grate the outside of the rind with the small holes of a cheese grater. Add the zest to sauces, desserts, or drinks. Orange zest is delicious on chocolate, in cranberry sauce, and on chicken. Lemon zest is also great on top of chicken or halibut, or sprinkled over vanilla cake frosting.

Dinner Parties

It's great to entertain and have friends over. If friends call to say they are heading by for an impromptu visit or playdate and your house isn't as clean as you would like it, don't panic. Focus on what they will see first. Dust the entranceway and sweep the welcome mat. Fluff the couch or chairs or wherever you think you might be sitting. Beautify your bathroom; all guests go there at some point, so take a second and wipe the counter and sink, dim the lights, and light a candle. In fact, if it's evening, dim the lights

> When you have guests, ordinary beverages like iced tea, lemonade, or water with sliced lemon and lime always make a better impression when they're served in an interesting decanter, pitcher, or glass milk jug. This is a simple way to bring a little class to your entertaining at virtually no extra cost or effort.

and light candles throughout the house. It adds charm, and everything just seems to look better in candlelight. Scented candles or diffusers are great because guests will notice the aroma the minute they walk in.

What makes the biggest impression is the way you react when friends arrive. A warm, enthusiastic greeting makes any guest feel special right off the bat. It's a great way to start the evening. So even if you are flustered, don't greet them with, "I've been running around all day and the place is a mess!" Go with, "Hi! We are so excited you're here!"

Home Safe Home

If you have toddlers, it is very likely your home resembles a maximum security prison. I actually had to ask a six-year-old how to open a toilet lock at a friend's house. Baby proofing has gone high tech and is nothing to take lightly. Accidents kill more children each year than disease and violence combined. It is estimated that 90 percent of these accidents are preventable. The best protection is prevention, and it is better to be proactive than reactive. Kimberlee Mitchell, the founder of Boo Boo Busters, is a leader in this field. She is a child safety expert who has baby proofed thousands of homes and is trusted by celebrities such as Britney Spears, Katie Holmes and Tom Cruise, Nadya Suleman (the "Octomom"), and many others. Visit her website, BooBooBusters.com, for tips and consultation information. Visit BabyProofingDirectory.com or IAFCS.org (the website of the International Association for Child Safety) to find a safety expert near you and to learn everything you can. SafeKids.org is another great resource.

When you are traveling, blue painter's tape can help baby proof a hotel room. Band-Aids can also be used as outlet covers. Rubber bands and hair ties as well as those trendy Livestrong bracelets work great on cabinet handles.

I could fill a whole book on tips to make your home safer. This section is not meant to scare you, just to help prepare you. Knowledge brings confidence. This is merely a reminder to do your research. And please, I urge you to get training in first aid and CPR. (Yes, I am certified!) You can find a class or a certified instructor at EnjoyCPR.com. Consider hosting a class with some friends in your home. I am a big believer in a kind of variation on Murphy's law: If you know how to do it, you won't need it. I hope that is true for every single person reading this book.

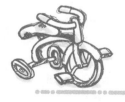

HERE ARE SOME QUICK SAFETY TIPS.

❀ Rule of thumb: Anything that can fit inside a toilet paper roll is a choking hazard.

❀ When little kids are around, use back burners and face pot handles in. (Keep in mind that children who play with pots and pans as toys may be more likely to try and reach for a pot or pan on a hot stove thinking it is his toy.)

❀ Install window guards with emergency release latches on all windows on the second floor or higher.

❀ Beware of toy stacking. Kids will pile up anything to get a view outside or to see over a deck railing.

❀ Anchor all items that are tipping hazards.

❀ Be aware of siblings accidentally leaving gates open or leaving small toy pieces around.

❀ Make sure smoke detectors are working. Keep spare packages of batteries in your junk drawer or tool box so you can replace dead batteries right away. The Vocal Smoke Alarm uses three different alarms to wake up your kids. It also allows you to record your own message using your kid's names and instructions on what to do if a fire breaks out.

❀ Store fire escape ladders in every bedroom on the second level and above.

❀ When your kids get older, have a calm meeting with the family to go over your plan for what to do in case of a fire, tornado, earthquake, hurricane, etc.— whatever is appropriate for where you live.

I do want to elaborate on water safety. Drowning is the leading cause of death for children under the age of five in California. And sadly, 69 percent of all swimming pool accidents happen when a parent is home. In 77 percent of those cases, the child had been seen five minutes or less before being missed or was thought to be taking a nap. It happens that quickly.

Kimberlee Mitchell's Safety Advice

1. Doors and gates leading to the pool area should be self-closing, locked, and alarmed.

2. Install a motion alarm in the pool and spa area.

3. Install a child-safe fence around the immediate pool area and/or install an approved pool cover. If you don't block off every access, the child will eventually find a way to get to the pool when you are not looking. Do not deceive yourself by thinking, "My child would never try that." Children are very smart and you must assume that a child will find a way to beat the system. If you do not, you are asking for trouble.

4. Use a wristband personal alarm with an in-house remote alarm, which lets you know if your child falls into the pool. The Safety Turtle is an ideal product for this last line of defense (SafetyTurtle.com).

5. When having a party, appoint a designated child watcher to constantly observe the children. Adults become preoccupied when they're socializing. They often assume someone else is watching the kids.

6. Do not consider children "water safe" just because they have had swimming lessons. THERE ARE NO WATER-SAFE CHILDREN. Kids lack the maturity level for sound judgment. Fun is their motivation, and a pool is fun. Unfortunately it is also dangerous.

7. No one should ever swim alone. Teach your children to use the buddy system. Since children learn by example, parents should follow these safety tips as well.

8. Toys and games should not be stored in or near the pool. The attraction of toys near the pool is much too inviting for children.

9. NEVER LEAVE CHILDREN UNATTENDED for any reason. Keep a cordless telephone near the pool at all times. A high percentage of child drownings occur when the children are left unattended while the caretaker answers the telephone, the front door, or while using the restroom.

10. If a child is missing, ALWAYS CHECK THE POOL FIRST! Don't assume you would have heard the child splash into the water. Time is critical; if the child has silently entered the water and is submerged, you have precious little time to react.

11. LEARN CPR. Everyone responsible for children, including grandparents, siblings, and babysitters, should know CPR. Post CPR instructions near the pool. Contact your local Red Cross for training information.

12. Common sense is the key to pool safety. There is no substitute for adult supervision.

Four-time Olympic gold medalist and eleven-time U.S. National Champion Lenny Krayzelburg shares the basics of water safety at home:

❀ Teaching kids to swim is critical. I always recommend swimming lessons, because children listen to experts and authority figures and it's sometimes tough for parents to teach water safety.

❀ Start teaching them before they're six months old. It is very womb-like in the water, and babies at this age are still comfortable on their backs. They also haven't developed fears yet.

❀ I teach kids the instinct to roll over onto their backs and breathe, which provides the ultimate tool for saving themselves if needed.

❀ When teaching the back float at home, position one hand underneath the back. Explain that this should be their automatic response for safety when in trouble in the water.

❀ I discourages floaties. They give kids a false sense of security and make them believe they can swim. Floaties also get kids into the bad habit of doggie paddling and keeping their head up to breathe, which can be very tiring should they ever fall in.

❀ Having a safety fence is important but it does not ensure your children's safety—you must also teach them how to swim and survive in the water.

Lenny Krayzelburg has taught thousands of kids to swim; for more information on his swim schools visit LennyKSwim.com.

Be Prepared

Cari Butler, the founder of the company Emergency Café (EmergencyCafe.com), offers kits for the home and the car to help you prepare for any situation.

One of the most important things you can have in your car is an emergency car hammer such as the Life-Hammer. It's a tool that can effortlessly cut a seatbelt and shatter a car window so you can escape from your car. It's small and costs less than $10. I keep mine in the glove box of my car. It is available at most hardware stores and all around on the Web.

First Aid Kits

You should have a first aid kit in your home and one in your car. Find prepackaged first aid kits from $3 to $100 at Target, Walmart, REI.com, Amazon.com, or RedCrossStore.org.

BloodStop gauze is a great addition to any medical kit. It stops the flow of blood in less than a minute. When blood hits it, the material turns to a gel that speeds co-agulation. It's good for deep cuts or nosebleeds.

Keep some emergency money—$20 or so—in your car for gas, parking, or any number of other unforeseen expenses. Hide some cash in the house as well; you never know when it will come in handy.

Wear Clean Underwear

Alexis Martin Neely's book *Wear Clean Underwear* is a must read. It helps guide you to the right legal decisions for your family while keeping things light and friendly. It is by far the easiest book to read on the heavy topic of how to make sure your children are taken care of if something happens to you. It is written in a narrative format and segmented into Choose Your Own Adventure–style scenarios with appropriate resources at the end.

My mom always told me to make sure I was wearing clean underwear when I left the house, in case I was in an accident. The first night I went out with my husband without our baby girl, I realized wearing clean underwear wasn't enough!

The entire night, I fretted and worried about my little girl at home without me. My mind inevitably strayed to what would happen to her, if something happened to us on the way home from dinner.

What I realized scared me to death. I was a lawyer and yet I hadn't put in place the planning necessary to make sure she'd be taken care of the right way if anything happened to us.

I'd left behind my cell phone number and my neighbor's phone number. It was only when we were sitting at dinner an hour away from home that I realized if something happened on the way home, my cell phone wouldn't work and my neighbor didn't have legal authority to take care of my baby.

The rest of the night was pretty much a bust. My poor husband.

After we got home, I put in place a plan to make sure there would never be a question about who should take care of my daughter or how she should be taken care of if anything happened to me and her dad.

When I found out that 69 percent of parents had never even named legal guardians for their children and that of the 31 percent who had, most had made at least one of six frequent mistakes, I knew I had to get parents the straight scoop on legal planning.

I've made it my mission to make great legal and financial advice accessible to parents so that no dad ever has to have their first date out with his wife after the baby is born ruined the way ours was by fear.

—Alexis Martin Neely, Hot Mom, lawyer, author, blogger, speaker, and legal expert

Switching gears to a lighter note, Most moms I know have one priority, making it through the day . . . as much as we try to be prepared as a parent, we all know there are so many variables, and when you are dealing with kids well . . . you just never know.

Grand-Mal Meltdown

My three-year-old, Rex, lost his mind the other night. We were at the end of what had been a lovely dinner party, fortunately in our own home. It started innocently enough: Dessert was distributed around the table and everyone was eating happily. On one side of me, my older boy, Mason, generously offered me a bite of his and I took him up on it. (I've been watching my waistline, so I didn't have a dessert of my own.) On the other side of me, cherubic little Rex sweetly asked, "Would you like a bite of mine?"

"Why, yes, I'd love a bite!" Now, you might know where this is going already, but I had no idea what fury would be unleashed when I chomped down on that chocolate ice cream bar. Yes, you guessed it—the child screamed bloody murder. In fact, his reaction was so alarming, everyone at the table thought he must have bitten his tongue or something. He screamed so loud and for so long, there were moments I thought we had better alert the authorities or call 9-1-1 or at least apologize to the neighbors.

After enduring enough of Rex's ear-blistering blast, the dinner guest politely excused themselves and my husband and I settled in to figure out what went wrong. We asked him over and over what happened, but he was too upset to talk. There was nothing we could do: We had to go about the evening, put Mason to bed, clean up the dishes, and call it a day—all the while trying to calm Rex and solve the mystery.

Finally, exhausted, he quieted down long enough to sniffle a few words, ones I'll never forget: "Your . . . sniff . . . bite . . . sniff, sniff . . . was too big." And there you have it, the maddening, unpredictable, mind-numbing impossibility that is parenting.

Why am I telling you all this? Well, it has been a few days now and Rex has recovered just fine. I, however, will never be the same. I mean, he is usually a reasonable child, so how would I know he would go off the deep end on this particular night? But shouldn't I have seen this coming? Why on earth did I take that bite? Why, God, why?

The truth is, there is so much of parenting that we just can't be prepared for. In the newborn days, it's the diaper blowouts that go all the way up the back of the baby's shirt, the spit-up all over you right before you are set to walk out the door, the projectile pee that douses the newly hung curtains, or even the realization that you haven't made eye contact with your spouse for a week.

It's a messy business indeed! As new moms all we can do is try to stay calm, talk to our friends, and try to learn from the experience.

—Abigail Tuller, editor in chief of
Pregnancy and *Mom* magazines

Seven

 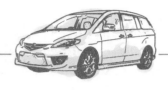

Rock That Minivan

My husband's idea of rough sex is when I don't shave my legs.
—Stephanie Blum, comedian and Hot Mom of three

A pound of tired, a pinch of hormones, and a sprinkle of over-whelm is a recipe for stress on any relationship. As women we are naturally maternal and those instincts will kick in big-time once your baby arrives. Your current baby (aka your hubby) will be feeling the hit. There are any number of reasons your relationship and sex life get more complicated after your baby is born. A variety of physical and hormonal factors can cause some women to lose their sex drive after giving birth. Lack of sleep can also contribute to a lack of interest or energy for sex for both new parents. Some men experience delivery room trauma, making it hard for them to see their wives as sexual beings, but in time most get over it, and your sex drive will come back.

Most women need emotional intimacy to as a prelude or precursor to sex. For most men, on the other hand, emotional intimacy comes from sex, so when the sex dries up, men tend to feel emotionally disconnected and may withdraw. When he's withdrawn, you may not feel the desire to be intimate, and so goes the vicious cycle.

There is no simple solution for everyone. You have to find what is going to fit for you two as a couple. Acknowledging that a healthy sex life is critical to a healthy relationship and making it a priority will help you make it happen.

Create a Sacred Space

Declare your bedroom a toy-free zone! As moms, our homes quickly become crowded with toys, swings, and the latest activity mats. It is very important to keep at least one room—your bedroom—as your sacred space, your sanctuary. It should be a husband and wife's bedroom, not a mom and dad's. It is hard to get physical if you have kids in the bed or if you are rolling over on action figures. This should be your room for making love, or just relaxing and reading together, or watching your favorite shows together—a place for bonding and intimacy that doesn't involved the kids. Claim that space. Put candles and flowers by the bed. Have photos of the two of you as a couple, not family or baby pictures, at least not in this room—they can be anywhere and everywhere else in the house, but this room should be designed to inspire romance and connection. I know it sounds corny, but believe me, it works; our environment sets the mood and can easily turn us on or turn us off.

Happy parents have an easier time raising happy children. For many parents, the only time they have to relax together, talk, or express love is at night after the kids go to sleep. If you make a habit of bringing the kids into bed with you, you will lose out on your special time together as a couple and as individuals. Sleeping in bed with you is not healthy for kids in the long run, either. What message are you sending to them? That they need you for everything. As parents we want to be there for our children, but in real life we can't be. We need to teach our children not just how to do things, but to do things on their own (like sleep in their own crib or bed). Look, I know how wonderful it feels to snuggle in bed with your child; it is one of my great pleasures. When a child is sick or a parent is out of town, I think it's fine for them to hop in bed with you, or as a treat. There are always exceptions. But if the exception becomes the rule, it can create problems down the road. Say it with me: happy parents have an easier time raising happy children. It is critical to claim time for yourselves each night and to claim your bedroom as your sacred space as a couple.

In the first few weeks home our new spawn refused to sleep anywhere but in bed with us. She was having none of the adorable bassinet decorated in the pink etoile I'd so carefully chosen. She screamed the second she was placed down onto its plush sixteenth of an inch of plastic padding, like she was being lowered onto hot coals, which inevitably forced us to bring her into our bed as a last-ditch option. Having a seven-pound baby in a bed with two adults is far from relaxing; it was like trying to snuggle with a Ming vase. We kept an all-night semiconscious vigil, petrified of falling fully asleep and mistakenly rolling over onto her . . . to be fair, some people who aren't me swear by the family bed. I think that's great if you can and want to sleep that way. But if I may say a word of caution: Once your child gets used to sleeping in your bed with you they won't want any part of their own room and own crib. So you need to be committed to doing the family bed at least until the baby's a teenager, or until it destroys your marriage.

—Stefanie Wilder-Taylor,
from *Sippy Cups Are Not for Chardonnay and Other Things I Had to Learn as a New Mom*

Play for the Same Team

We all want to be good parents, and want to know and do everything possible to take the best care of our newborns, but it is equally important that we remember to direct some of that energy into taking care of and nurturing our relationships with our partners. It is important that you bring the baby into YOUR loving relationship, making you all a unit, not the two of you directing your energy to the baby.

There is a big difference that is crucial in preserving your family unit. You have to be on the same team. You will have different parenting styles or decisions now and then, but in general remain a united front. If your husband tells the kids no and you tell them yes, it emasculates him. (I'm looking at you, Kate Gosselin.) This also signals to the kids that one of you is dominant and that they can divide you. They need to see you two as a team. Remember, you are doing this for the sake of your children; you are modeling relationships for them. Their future relationships will most likely mirror yours. They deserve to be a part of that same loving union that brought them into the world. So stick together, be a team, have respect for your husband as a parent and a decision maker.

More Dates, Fewer Diapers

Good ol' date night—I wish I had some fancy or unique spin on this, but the truth is, setting time aside at least once a week to go on a date or to have quality one-on-one time together is important and has been proven to work. I add that you are absolutely NOT allowed to talk about the baby during your date.

No exceptions!

Date night doesn't have to always be some big romantic event. Sometimes it's just nice to unwind and talk to each other without interruption. Create a candlelit dinner after the kids have gone to bed, put on your favorite music, sit on your front porch.

If going out isn't always practical, planning dinners and time together at home can be fun and romantic, too.

> *Dating your man is a great way to keep it HOT! Dinners at a new spot or just meeting for a drink before you go home to the kids can keep the desire alive.*
> —Keisha Whitaker,
> Hot Mom of three and wife of actor Forest Whitaker

It was very hard for me to leave my kids. It was just devastating to have to get a babysitter that wasn't family. But when you find that right person, to still be willing to go out to dinner and not lose your relationship with your husband . . . that was work for me. I was like, "I love you and all, honey, but I'm busy. I got my babies!"

Pete was like, "Oh my God, I'll fly your mom down! Can we just spend the night, one night somewhere?" So I said, "Okay, sure."

You have to stay connected to each other. I know my husband felt not so much a part of it and [when he felt] not a part of me, it made everything so much harder. That was a lesson that took me a while to learn.

—Bridgette Wilson Sampras

Have a Night in Italy

Make homemade pasta or pizza, open a Chianti, serve some gelato for dessert, pick an Italian-themed movie—*Life is Beautiful, The Italian Job, Roman Holiday*, or even *My Cousin Vinny*.

This works equally for a night in France, Mexico, Japan, India, etc. Get creative!

BABY ON A BUDGET

Eating out can get pricey. If you need a change of atmosphere, go out *after* dinner. Eat with the kids, then go out for drinks and some dancing afterward.

Romance at Home

When the kids are asleep, set up some candles, dim the lights, put on soft music, and schedule a couples massage. Many spas offer in-home massage services.

Or treat each other to a massage, but go all out—get some nice scented oil, put towels in the dryer to make them nice and warm, and lay them over each other before you start the massage.

Skinny dip. If you have a pool, there is nothing like the feeling of splashing around in the water nude late at night. Removing your suits adds an element of excitement.

House-sit for someone with a fabulous place—hopefully a friend or relative with a nice view and a fireplace or a big pool or Jacuzzi. Being someplace new can feel fresh and exciting.

Wear a sexy nightie or pajamas, cuddle in bed or on the couch, and watch romantic movies together. This always sets the mood.

HERE ARE A FEW OF MY FAVORITE SEXY, ROMANTIC MOVIES AND MOVIES WITH GREAT LOVE SCENES.

✿ The Bridges of Madison County

✿ Bridget Jones's Diary

✿ Bull Durham

✿ Dirty Dancing

❀ *Ghost*

❀ *Love Actually*

❀ *The Notebook*

❀ *An Officer and a Gentleman*

❀ *Once*

❀ *Pretty Woman*

❀ *Risky Business*

❀ *Shakespeare in Love*

❀ *Titanic*

❀ *When Harry Met Sally*

Date Night Times Two

I love going out with other fun couples, and yes, it still counts as a date night if another couple is involved. It's social adult time that you spend together. Just be sure to choose people who are fun and uplifting and who have a great relationship. Find a couple you both like to spend time with. You can also order in and plan game nights at your home. Playing on the same team together is great for laughs and for bonding. I personally love Boggle and Taboo.

Day Dates

If the kids are at Grandma's and you have a Sunday afternoon free, get dressed up and go to open houses in wealthy neighborhoods. It's fun to look and imagine.

Take him on a surprise date. Blindfold him, take him in the car, and bring him somewhere he has been wanting to go—maybe a baseball game, a hike, sailing lessons, a new restaurant, a picnic, a movie he has been dying to see. The element of mystery will make the destination and the date that much more fun.

Fantasize and Surprise

Sex isn't the only way to connect with your partner. Fantasizing and surprising one another can cement bonds and create deeper intimacy. I know it seems impossible to be flirty when you are exhausted and busy feeding and changing a newborn every few hours, but it only takes a minute to write an enticing note or to leave a sultry message on his phone or nightstand. Arousal and intimacy start in the mind, so get his wheels turning. Anticipation is a HUGE turn-on. It's not as hard as you think. Little things really do mean a lot and go a long way. Grab his butt when the kids aren't looking. Smile a sexy, naughty smile when he least expects it. Touch his arm affectionately when you walk by.

Try sending him a sexy card in the mail. Write a love note and hide it in a book he's reading. Call him on the phone and sing a silly love song. Make up the words. Sing out of tune. It will only take a few minutes and will definitely put a smile on his face. Put dirty (or sweet) Post-it notes about how sexy he is and how much he turns you on, in places where only he'll find them. Surprise him by putting a thong or some other suggestive item in his briefcase. Call him home from work because you want to make love to him so badly you can't take it. Spray just a tiny bit of your fragrance on his briefcase so he has the scent of you all day. Use your lipstick to leave him a sultry message on the bathroom mirror.

Flash him a sweet and sexy smile when he least expects it, or just flash him for fun! Igniting the passion really is just as easy as touching him affectionately when you walk by or giving him a quick pat on the butt. Get creative! Come up with special code words that mean "I want you!" for when the kids or relatives are around. Instead of a peck on the cheek, surprise him with a sensual kiss as he heads out the door. It can literally change the mood of the entire day. It really is the little things that build intimacy and ignite passion. Everyone wants to feel desired, even men.

Fais-Moi un Bisou

Kiss: (v) To touch or caress with the lips as an expression of affection, respect, or amorousness.

Kissing is a bonding behavior, the affirmation of attachment. Kissing can and should be tremendously intimate. Not to mention that our lips have gobs of sensory receptors, making the intensity of kissing somebody you care about deliciously meaningful and dizzying. Need more reasons to start your day off with a good, solid, tongue-tangling French kiss? Well, there are many health benefits of kissing, too. It reduces stress. When you kiss, you breathe deeper. Kissing actually produces a lot of the physiological changes that meditation produces. Kissing can help increase the levels of oxytocin and endorphins, which reduces anxiety, quiets your mind, and simply makes you feel good. Kissing is good for oral hygiene as it stimulates saliva flow, which can wash bacteria off your teeth and help bring plaque levels down to normal. Kissing is also said to burn calories and boost immunity. I just know it's fun, and a "peck" to me feels obligatory like a semi-romantic handshake. Taking a minute to extend a soft, gentle, passionate kiss can have you thinking about each other all day. Kissing someone you love makes you feel happy, and when our sense of well-being improves our self-esteem increases. We feel more secure and better about ourselves, and our outer persona reflects it. The ladies at Mommy and Me won't be able to help but notice.

> *Kissing is passion and romance and what keeps people together.*
> —William Cane, author of *The Art of Kissing*

> *Kissing is a means of getting two people so close together that they can't see anything wrong with each other.*
> —Rene Yasenek

Create a Kiss Trap

Do you miss mistletoe 364 of the 365? Make a year-round kiss-on-demand substitute. Grab a foam heart at the craft store. Decorate it with feathers and tie a card to it

Love Sneak Attacks

When people feel appreciated they are more likely to extend appreciation in return. It's a good cycle to keep going in any home and in any relationship. As busy as we might be, taking a minute or two here and there to leave a sexy note with lipstick on the bathroom mirror or hiding a sexy Post-it note in his sock drawer can reap you benefits worth a hundred times the effort. So create a "love arsenal" for sneak attacks. Stash a box and fill it with his favorite candies, funny or romantic cards, anything that has meaning to you both. This way when you are feeling sweet or wanting him to feel appreciated you can leave the candies and notes on his pillow, in his briefcase, in the glove box of his car, in his raincoat pocket, or in the book he's reading—anywhere he might stumble upon it. The romantic quotient is turned up a notch when someone finds or gets something unexpected. Love notes and messages are easy to create and the impact is always greater if it's hidden and found at a random time or place.

As busy moms we rarely have time to run out and get a card or his favorite treat on a whim, so have a stash on hand for when the mood strikes you and you are feeling flirty and cheeky. A great time to stock up is actually after Valentine's day, when everything is 50 percent to 75 percent off.

Sidewalk chalk is another way to leave a sweet note. Let the kids make drawings, but you can write a message to greet your honey when he gets home. Glow-in-the-dark chalk is also available; having a cute message on the driveway or walkways is a fun way to greet him when he arrives from a late trip or night at the office.

Sex and the New Parent

Babies no doubt change the quantity of sex and the quality, but Hot Moms have GREAT SEX! Why? When you are confident and empowered, and when your inner goddess is tended to and unleashed, you feel desirable and you create natural desire. A healthy sex life directly affects your family. It's no secret that sexually satisfied people are happier and more optimistic. Sex can transform and increase your overall energy and vitality. Sex is a crucial element of your relationship. It bonds you; it is the act of giving yourself completely to another. We are designed for sex. Sex triggers extremely strong emotions. If you are not having sex you are missing out.

The more you love yourself and the more confident you feel, the easier this will be. Exercise your sensuality and passion regularly. How does this make you a better mom? A night of great sex can carry your mood throughout the whole day. Feeling love and giving love only strengthens your relationship, and your mood and your relationship DIRECTLY affect your kids.

A Dad's View of Post-Baby Sex

Sex after pregnancy is a topic that needs a great deal of consideration, exploration, and debate. If there is one thought in that vacuous mind of his, it's sex. He's a man; he's capable of thinking about sex during a funeral, a football game, or during dinner at your parents' house. It's not like he can control the sex part of his brain . . . it's been poorly wired by evolution, and no amount of Darwinian evolutionary mumbo jumbo is likely to change that.

If there is ever a time in your relationship when your sexual timetables clash, it's going to be the first twelve to twenty-four months after the baby is born. Like two out-of-control trains traveling aimlessly on the subway, you may not ever enter the same terminal at the same time unless you get to the control panel and start fiddling with the levers.

I don't think there is a definitive answer as to whether women have an increased or decreased sexual appetite after pregnancy. Tiredness and sheer exhaustion aside, it would seem that there are periods of "don't come near me" and "I'm a raging nymphomaniac" with relatively calm times in between.

I'm not qualified or stupid enough to try and coach women through their sexuality issues . . . after all, I'm no Dr. Phil or Jerry Springer, but I can help you out when it comes to your man. Whether it's keeping him at bay but happy when you're not interested or getting him on the job when you are dying for it, you can keep your relationship in good shape.

Let's explore the complex sexual issues that arise after the birth so that you can enjoy your celibacy in peace or orgasm to your heart's content.

Is he a Can or a Can Not?

We've interviewed hundreds of men across the nation for our Being Dad films and it doesn't matter what color, religion, or creed they are, some men can have sex after pregnancy and some can't.

The everyday Joes fit into one of two categories:

Sex after baby offers no issues and they are bang up for it, as always.

While still finding their partner sexy, they lose their mojo.

The big questions about sex and pregnancy is, is your man a can or a can not? What can you do if your sex drives aren't in sync? How can you penetrate his gray matter to pull in the reins or re-ignite his mojo?

Sex and intimacy are an important part of relationships, and a degradation of the sexual relationship can cause emotional issues in both you and your man unless you can communicate on the subject and work through issues as they arise, or don't arise as the case may be.

The can-do man is up for it, day or night, all the way up to the birth and after the birth, which is terrific if you actually have a sex drive but a nightmare if sex is the last thing on your mind. Don Juan or I Really Don't Juan . . . it's a fine line.

Sex, as you know it, will change for the next few years. You'll have less time, be more tired, and genuinely despise each other for short periods of time . . . sounds sexy, doesn't it.

If he's doing something wrong, let him know. If it's something completely unrelated to him, explain the problem so he doesn't feel detached from you. If he's pouting over not getting any and thinking that it's the beginning of the end, then problems may arise.

Of course, there may be physical reasons that you are unable to have sex, and you shouldn't feel guilty for not wanting it or not being able to have it. Communication is the key, and as long as he knows your reasons and how you feel, chances are he will be understanding.

The tendency for my fellow man (everyone except for me, that is . . .) is to either pout if they are not getting enough or withdraw if they are feeling sexually insecure. You need to be mindful of each other's fears and concerns, open about your feelings, and hopefully your ying and his yang can get in sync.

Let's face it, sex is terrific and the best fun you can have for free. Over the next few years it will be easy to let your sex life slide or become non-existent. While we haven't conducted any formal studies on the matter, it stands to reason that maintaining a good, healthy sex life can be nothing but beneficial. Your relationship is paramount; if sex has been a part of that relationship before kids, then it will need to be post-kids. Sure, there are millions of reasons and excuses not to have sex and it's easier not to, but find the time; the dishes and dirty nappies will still be there when you've finished!

—Troy Jones, director of Being Dad USA
(BeingDadUSA.com)

The Most Common Reasons Women Don't Have Sex

Excuse #1: Too Tired

Is "tired" the new headache? Exhaustion is a legitimate reason, but putting sex off for later can easily become never. Start examining why you are so tired and find ways to alleviate some of the workload. Take naps when the kids nap, buy the brownies instead of making them, set a strict bedtime for the kids, stop being Superwoman. You may be surprised to hear it, but sex actually energizes you. Touch and massage are incredibly powerful turn-ons. If you are too tired, learn how to massage and relax one another. Sensual rubbing after a long day, with the right oils and techniques, could be something you look forward to. Intimacy is whatever you make it or want it to be, so create loving rituals together. Not to rub salt in the we're-not-having-enough-sex wound, but I know plenty of couples who have great sex lives—exhausted or not. In fact, they have more sex when they are tired because it's their way of relaxing and feeling good—sex floods the brain with endorphins and oxytocin, which makes you both feel wonderful.

> *Motherhood and sex have a lot in common. When they're great, they're really great. When they're monotonous, or downright disagreeable, you can be sure that most people are not going to admit to it."*
> —Valerie Davis Raskin, *Great Sex for Moms*

Solution: Choreplay.

If all of your responsibilities are taking their toll and your sex life is suffering, talk to your husband about it. If relieving you of some of the chores that are making you so tired will make you more willing and able in bed, I am sure he will gladly oblige! Many women have actually said that it turns them on when their man helps out around the house. Use the reward system, ladies; it works with your pets and your kids and it will work with your man. If your husband does something well, praise him. If he swaddles a baby like no other, let him know and be sure to brag about it in front of other people. This will make him feel capable and respected and more willing to help in other areas with the kid.

If he empties the dishwasher or cooks a nice meal, tell him how amazing he is and give him the type of reward you know will get him excited. This will only encourage him to help you out more often and will create a positive cycle and foundation for a happy home. Happy parents have an easier time raising happy kids.

> I find that the more we indulge in quickies, the easier it is to build the fire in our more extended sexual routine and awaken the passion and frenzy we had in the early days of dating—before kids, mortgages, stress, bills, and a far more complicated life. My first thought after our little rendezvous is always "Why don't we do this more often?"
>
> —Hot Mom of two

Excuse #2: No Time

Solution: Make the time.

The bottom line is, we ALWAYS find time to do the things we really want to do. If you want to make love to your partner, then turn off the TV, put the kids to bed earlier, and do it. Claim the nights. Except for special occasions, my son is in bed no later than 8:30, without fail. The nights are mine. Check your schedule and see where you can reorganize to fit in more "play" time for yourself. Wake up a half hour before the kids do. We seem to have no problem finding reasons or excuses why we CAN'T. Here is a short list of why you CAN.

- ❀ The kids are at your mom's.

- ❀ It's date night.

- ❀ You just hit rewind on the *Toy Story* video.

- ❀ You've still got it.

- ❀ The sleepover is not at your house.

- ❀ Your pre-pregnancy jeans actually fit.

- ❀ Your husband wants you badly.

- ❀ Because you are totally turned on.

- ❀ *Modern Family* is a rerun.

- ❀ Your child is at soccer practice for an hour.

- ❀ Your new attitude turns him on more than ever.

Take responsibility for your sex life. If you are not having great sex, or not having sex at all, ask yourself why. YOU have the power to change it. If it's been a while, you just have to retrain. The more sex appeal you give off, the more your partner will respond to you. Start building the desire again. Surprise him with all you have discovered about yourself and have him come home to a candlelit house one night

I blame my mother for my poor sex life. All she told me was, "The man goes on top and the woman underneath." For three years my husband and I slept in bunk beds.

—Joan Rivers

after work. It's not practical all the time, but make arrangements for someone to watch the kids now and then. Pencil in special nights for just you two. Don't let it get away from you; it's so easy to fall into the rut. Call it date night, call it booty night, call it whatever you like. Get creative, be fun, be spontaneous.

Solution #2: Make mine a quickie.

I have heard quickies referred to as the light snack of sex. Quickies are underrated. In my opinion they are a necessary function in any relationship. They're spontaneous and fun when mixed in with a healthy lovemaking routine—and hey, if it's done right, you can fit an orgasm right in between a commercial break!

Excuse #3: Not in the Mood

Abstinence does not make the loins grow fonder. Sex is a vital part of a healthy, loving relationship, and it's important to devote time and energy to intimacy. Many women are very skilled at denying its significance. It's no secret or surprise that your sex drive can lessen after kids, but if you are not hot for him at all, you have a problem. The fact that you are rarely interested in sex or are zoned out thinking about little Johnnie's preschool

You know that look women get when they want sex? Me neither!
—Drew Carey

application during a rendezvous could be a sign that you are too caught up with your responsibilities as mom to feel sexually desirable. When you stop having sex, your natural testosterone levels lower. The best way to increase your desire for sex is actually to have more sex.

It's a safe bet that what's going on in your sex life is

a very good indicator of what's going on in your marriage. You can't be passionate about your partner if you are not passionate about yourself and your desirability. Sex builds confidence and a sense of well-being in both of you. One of the most loving things you can do is to pursue your husband sexually. Make sure your husband goes to sleep with a smile on his face; he will wake up thinking he is the luckiest man in the world and he will be excited to come home to you. Bottom line: If you make time for sex, you will feel more connected, your attitude will be more willing, and your husband will be eternally grateful. You are doing this for yourself as much as for your husband. A man who is respected, needed, and fulfilled will knock down doors for you.

The food you eat and the things you read and watch can help you feel more excited about sex and romance.

Solution #1: Here are some foods that will help boost your libido.

❀ Oysters are a well-known aphrodisiac. The secret could be their high levels of zinc and dopamine.

❀ Chocolate contains phenylethylamine, which stimulates the release of hormones that make you feel like you are in love. It's also fun for sex play; drizzle some on your man.

❀ Garlic contains allicin, an ingredient that increases blood flow to the sexual organs. (Just stock up on breath mints, too.)

Solution #2: Read romance novels.

I know this may sound silly but read romance novels. Reading about sexy romantic encounters can help spark your imagination!

Bedtime Stories to Get You H-O-T

If your schedule is anything like mine, then the last thing you probably read was the label of the children's Tylenol bottle. Reading has become sort of an ancient art. Reading anything other than a set of instructions for a kid's toy, a recipe, or the contents of your Tucks wipes while you're sitting on the shitter is a complete luxury. And if you are able to pick up the relic called a "novel" or "memoir," you end up having to read them a paragraph at a time, which doesn't bode well for actually finishing anything but the back matter in the next century. So it shouldn't be a surprise that moms are reaching for a different kind of book these days—the erotic romance novel.

These books are a cheap grocery store romance novel and full-blown erotica hybrid, and offer moms a decent plot and fairly hot sex, all in under fifty thousand words.

And it'll probably only take you about a thousand to get off.

Yep, these puppies are steamier than anything you've probably ever gotten your hands on, without being blatantly pornographic, and some are written by authors who are moms themselves! These books are well-written erotic stories with character development and way more than just the stereotypical romantic trysts. Think soap opera with sex. Pretty freaking hot sex, actually. Combine that with intelligent writing and you've got the perfect recipe for moms—stimulation for the mind and the muff. Erotic romance novels take what's generally missing for women in porn and apply it to something you can stick in your diaper bag or nightstand stable, or even better, download right to your Kindle, computer, or iPod.

Aside from the satisfaction you'll get from actually finishing something other than your kid's dinner plates, they're the perfect length for in between naps, feedings, or right before you hit the sack—talk about redefining the bedtime story.

And "I read a book last night" sounds way better than "I watched a porno"—at least at your neighborhood playgroup, anyway.

—Kristen Chase,
author of *The Mominatrix's Guide to Sex*

Excuse #4: You Just Don't Feel Sexy

Solutions: Turn off the cartoons and turn on yourself!

Sexiness is wanting to feel desired and being desired. It is hard to feel sexy when you are changing stinky diapers all day, running on only a few hours of sleep, and showering so quickly the mirror doesn't even fog. Just as these aspects of our lives affect our sexuality, our sexuality affects every other part of our lives. It affects your happiness, your energy, and your confidence as a mother and a woman. That's right—you are still a woman! It is sometimes easy to forget that and let the feminine, sexy side of yourself slide. That is why is it so important to nurture every part of who you are, including that sexy inner siren. Think you don't have an "inner siren," that sexy, sultry woman inside you? EVERY woman has an inner goddess. She may be buried under clothes you pulled from the hamper, but I promise, she's in there, and it's time to wake her up and let her loose! I promise, your attitude about sex is more important than the size of your waist, breasts, thighs, or butt. It's about presentation. Work your assets and feel confident.

There exists in every woman a hidden erotic creature, a center of sexual power and self-knowledge. She's the wild, feline, untamed part of you, your sexual alter ego—and the opposite of the "good girl." By nature, women are sensual beings. Our breasts protrude, our butts stick out, our hips curve, and our waists indent. Many of us have been conditioned to hide or diminish our sexuality . . . Get to know your inner erotic creature. Who is she? She is different for every woman. For you she might be a playful 1940s pinup, a Montana cowgirl, a pretty-in-pink baby doll, a black-leather-clad rocker

chick, a bespectacled librarian, a French
maid, or an elegant Park Avenue seductress.
At times she may be a combination of many
different things. Your erotic creature has
moods that evolve over time and defy simple
labels. She's as idiosyncratic as you are.
—Sheila Kelley, creator of the S Factor

The more comfortable you are with your own sexuality, the more sexy you will feel, and the more sexy you
will be. It all starts in you. The more capable you are of
truly loving yourself, the more loving you will feel, and
the more loving you will be. So let go of all those fears
and insecurities and inhibitions. Who said that moms
shouldn't be sexy? We've been so conditioned to believe
that once you become "mom," that sexual creature
inside of you is no longer appropriate. Being a mother
only adds to your sex appeal. Your capacity for love and
caring are stronger and greater than ever. Turn some of
that love toward yourself. Commit to dusting off your
inner goddess and letting her shine.

Just as the everyday aspects of our lives affect our
sexuality (staying up all night with the baby, running
around to soccer practice and activities all day), our
sexuality affects every other part of our lives (our happiness and our energy and our confidence, and our relationship with our partner, to name a few). Like anything
worthwhile, we must make it a priority. Dedicate time
each week to nurturing that sensual, beautiful woman
inside of you, then start dedicating some time each day.

In order to really feel sexy and empowered, you need to lose any inhibitions you have with your body. A good understanding of and connection with your body is essential to emotional happiness and sexual health. Love your body. The next time you are in the shower, acknowledge your curves, the definition in your arms . . . really work on appreciating how beautiful you are. Will you do me a favor? Every time you take a shower, as your lather the soap around your body, repeat these words: "My body is more beautiful than ever. I am a sexy, sensual woman." If you do this every day, your body will respond to this appreciation and you will grow increasingly more beautiful, inside and out. The effects of loving your body will truly astound you.

Doing sexy things will also help unleash your inner siren . . .

The Scent of a Woman: Create a Signature Scent

Scent is a powerful thing. It arouses people on the primal level. The nose can pinpoint up to ten thousand smells. What is your signature scent for romance? If you don't have one, find one. Talk to your partner about what his favorite scents are or go shopping together. Choose something that makes you feel sexy when you smell it. Wear this when you are in the mood, as a signal to him. Wear it when you make love. It won't be long before he associates the slightest whiff of this scent with the pleasure of your rendezvous, so spraying only a tiny amount on his jacket or briefcase can make him fantasize about you all day.

A few scents that most men love are vanilla, cinnamon, and lavender. Cleopatra used lavender to seduce many men.

BABY ON A BUDGET

Love Spell body mists from Victoria's Secret are just that—and cost only $9 for a large 8.4 ounce bottle.

Auric Blends Egyptian Goddess roll-on oil smells fantastic and drives men wild. It can be found at Whole Foods and various drug stores for only $4 to $7 (or at AuricBlends.com). This is a light musk for those who want a subtle, non-fruity scent.

$TUFF TO DROOL OVER

Mix your own signature scent. Mémoire Liquide, which is favored by celebs such as Kate Hudson and Reese Witherspoon, offers its custom-made scents at Studio Beautymix at Fred Segal in Santa Monica and Blooming dale's at Fifty-ninth Street in New York City. You can also choose from a selection of ready-to-wear fragrances at Henri Bendel. The fragrances start at $45 for one-quarter ounce.

Bad-Girl Panties

A little lingerie can spice up your love life, especially after maternity underwear has become a staple. Men are visually stimulated, and lingerie is a turn-on for your man, but it should also make you feel feminine, womanly, and beautiful. Garter belts are super sexy. Wear them in bed, or on a date night— then surprise him by sliding his hand up your dress until he realizes you are wearing no ordinary pantyhose!

If, like most new moms, you start to feel a little self-conscious about your body

I answered the phone one night to a crank call: "What are you wearing?" he said. I said, "My MATERNITY UNDERWEAR!" He hung up. I called back and got his machine.

—Stephanie Blum, comedian and Hot Mom of three

after baby, keep in mind that confidence is your sexiest weapon. Own the fact that you are fabulous and a Hot Mom no matter what your new shape is. We are our own worst critics. The more comfortable you are with yourself, the sexier you will feel and the sexier you will be. Sexy doesn't have to mean lingerie; it's anything that helps you get in touch with the woman inside of you. It could mean red lipstick, a manicure, or a hot bath to make you feel sensual. Sexy is an attitude and a feeling. It all starts with you. As a mom, your capacity for love and care will be stronger than ever, so don't forget to turn a little of that love toward yourself. Take a trip to the lingerie store and buy outrageous panties—maybe a bright red or hot pink, something out of character for you—then surprise your husband, or wear them to your next PTA meeting just for fun. No one will see them, but you will instantly feel sexier and more daring. Every mom should have at least one bra and panty set that isn't practical but makes her feel gorgeous and sensual. Every mom should also have a seductive outfit—your LBD of lingerie. I always recommend baby-doll dresses because they are flattering on almost every figure and they are very forgiving if you still have some baby weight to lose.

THESE ARE SOME OF MY FAVORITE LINGERIE BRANDS.

✿ Cosabella (Cosabella.com)

✿ Hanky Panky (HankyPanky.com)

✿ NancyMeyer.com (an online retailer that has an assortment of lingerie, loungewear, and sleepwear by high-end designers)

✿ On Gossamer (OnGossamer.com)

✿ Wendy Glez (WendyGlez.com)

BABY ON A BUDGET

Victoria's Secret has a wide variety of sexy lingerie. If you don't have time to stop in to a store near you, browse through the pages and pages of baby-doll dresses they have online (VictoriasSecret.com) starting at around $30. Check their website often, because they also have incredible sales!

AgentProvocateur.com has some of the most gorgeous, well-made, and sexiest lingerie on the market. Bras start at $150, and slips and nighties range from $290 to $500.

High Chairs and High Heels

Nothing makes me feel sexier then when I am rocking a great pair of heels. It's true it is just a pair of shoes, but heels can change your entire look. Besides making you appear taller, they accentuate the appearance of your calves and cause your legs to look longer. Heels make you look slimmer and more feminine as you walk because your hips swing and your back arches and your butt and chest are forced out. Some woman could run a marathon in high heels, but if you are no Carrie Bradshaw in that department, don't worry; wear only what you're comfortable in and makes you feel good. Maybe keep an open mind and buy a fun pair just for the bedroom.

Cole Haan has teamed up with Nike to create some of the most innovative and comfy high heels available today. The heels utilize Nike Air technology to cushion the ball and heel of the foot. They have edgy and modern designs and colors, and prices range from $79.95 (on sale) to $348. Go to ColeHaan.com and search for the Air collection.

Designer Michael Kors launched his Michael by Michael Kors collection, which looks upscale, with his impeccable taste and design, but is more reasonably priced. (You can find a sexy Michael by Michael Kors heel for around $100.) The line is available at department stores such as Nordstrom and Macy's.

BABY ON A BUDGET

Michael Antonio's heels have been featured in *People* magazine's style watch, as well as many other magazines. His heels are on trend, and are very affordable at $39 to $70 a pair. Go to MichaelAntonio.com to view the collection and to find retailers.

Sites like Bluefly.com offer designer shoes and heels at up to 80 percent off. Shoes.com has a huge selection from a variety of top designers and also runs great sales.

$TUFF TO DROOL OVER

Yves Saint Laurent's heels are a celebrity favorite and sell for around $700 a pair (YSL.com).

Christian Louboutin shoes, with their signature red soles, are a staple on the red carpet. Shoes start at about $500 and range upward to more than $2,000 a pair.

Couture.Zappos.com has wide selection of designer shoes sure to fit any style.

Love Songs

Jump on iTunes and make a sexy CD—something guaranteed to get you in the mood. Some of my romantic favorites are Sade, Michael Bublé, Chris Isaak, Norah Jones, and Ray LaMontagne.

Light My Fire

Candles are a great way to set a romantic mood or ambiance. They create a sense of warmth and elegance. The mixture of beautiful scents and soft lighting is a powerfully sexy combination. Use *un*scented candles during a meal so the smell doesn't interfere with the food you are about to enjoy. (Always remember to blow out the candles. I actually always use a candle snuffer, and I always make sure the candles are nestled safely in holders or glass jars.)

My favorite candle brands are Voluspa (Voluspa Candles.com) and Illume (IllumeCandles.com). Illume offers a His & Hers collection and a prepackaged group of "Quickies" votives for travel or love on the go.

BABY ON A BUDGET

If I want to really make an impact with a lot of candles, I often stock up at Ikea. They have candles in various colors from $1.99 and twelve-packs of tiny candles for $5.99.

$TUFF TO DROOL OVER

DayNa Decker (DayNaDecker.com) Couture Luxury Candles use botanical wax and patented Eco Wood wicks and come in sophisticated black boxes. Their medium size runs about $64 and large candles start at $92.

CandleLuxury.com offers a selection of high-end beautifully scented candles.

Conventional candles are made of petroleum-based paraffin wax, synthetic dyes, and artificial fragrances, which are toxic to produce and can result in indoor air pollutants. Cheaper wicks may contain traces of heavy metals, which may be released into the air during combustion. Soy wax is made from soybeans, is renewable, burns cleaner, and is said to last three times longer than paraffin wax.

HERE ARE SOME SOURCES FOR NATURAL ALTERNATIVES TO CONVENTIONAL CANDLES.

❀ BsaB bamboo candles (BsaBCandles.com) come in stylish bamboo pillars that can be refilled. They use 100 percent soy wax, cotton wicks, and essential oils.

❀ Paddywax candles (Paddywax.com) are beautifully packaged and make gorgeous gifts. They offer both soy wax and beeswax candles.

❀ Vermont-based Way Out Wax (WayOutWax .com) offers 100 percent soy candles that come in recycled glass and are scented with your choice of pure essential oils, with no artificial ingredients.

❀ If you want the romantic scent but don't like to have candles around, scent diffusers can make any rooms instantly smell great. I love Votivo diffusers. They come in so many delicious varieties (Votivo.com).

❀ Febreze Home Collection No Spill Wood Diffuser is perfect if you have lots of little hands around. It gives off a nice smell without any mess. Go to Febreze.com to find a retailer.

Think Outside the Bedroom

We are so conditioned to stay in the comfort zone. But Hot Moms aren't afraid to stay open to the erotic possibilities of the world around them. Open your mind—take a belly dancing class or try strip aerobics. Read erotic books and watch erotic movies. Most people find it exciting, although they are often reluctant to admit it. Visit a novelty shop, either with your lover or your girlfriends, and familiarize yourself with what's out there. You'll have a few laughs, maybe even get turned on. Just think outside the box: Create a sexy alter ego, with a name and everything, and let that erotic creature do the shopping! For fun, purchase something you never thought you would. You won't know whether you'll enjoy it until you've tried it, and who knows, it could add a new dimension to your sex life, alone or with a lover.

Repeat After Me: "I Am a Goddess in Bed"

We've already established that you can be a mom *and* a sex kitten. Confidence in yourself, in your body, and in your abilities will help you surrender to the moment, let go of your inhibitions, and be open and connected to your partner. Here are some tips to help you get started.

❀ Find new and interesting places to make love—a secluded area in your yard, even just on the floor or in the guest bedroom. It will add excitement and spontaneity. It's okay if you have a minivan; just make it rock now and then! Jump in that oh-so-convenient third row and make out like teenagers.

❀ Explore new positions. (I highly doubt you have done it *all*.) There are some great books, like the *Kama Sutra*; grab one and flip through it together.

❀ Blindfold your partner, and then have him blindfold you. When you take away the sense of sight, you heighten the sense of touch. Caress his skin with a feather or a silk scarf. Put a few peppermint breath mints in your mouth, get it nice and tingly, and then kiss him all over.

❀ Strip for each other. Now that you have your sexy lingerie, work it! Show it off and strut your stuff.

❀ Keep eye contact with your lover the entire time you make love.

❀ Take charge! Channel your inner dominatrix: Order him to kiss your toes, your knees, your inner thighs, and then . . .

❀ Send your man an e-mail with links to three pairs of high heels you like. Tell him to pick one pair and have it sent to you. When it arrives, meet him at the door wearing nothing but the heels.

❀ Take a bath together. Spread out some candles, put on that sexy CD you made, and soak in a nice tub.

❀ Sometime when you really don't want to make love, do it anyway.

❀ Sometime when you really do want to make love, don't—hold off.

❀ Every once in a while, wake your partner up in the middle of the night to make love.

❀ Write a love note in lipstick on your stomach or cleavage.

❀ Every year on your anniversary, decorate your car like a newlywed's, with shaving cream and dragging cans, then ride around all day. The kids will have a blast helping you decorate, and they'll get a kick out of driving around like that.

✿ If you're tech savvy, put a sexy ringtone or song on your man's cell phone and assign it to your number so that every time you call, he'll hear it. This will not only make him smile but will also make him subconsciously associate you with fun and sex, not just with being a mom.

✿ Send your man a special gift every day for the twelve days leading up to Christmas, each with a little note that begins, "On the first day of Christmas, my true love sent to me . . ." Every day's gift should be something sweet or something naughty: two champagne glasses, three thong undies . . . You get the idea.

Know where your hot spots are. Maybe you are turned on by a loving caress on your cheek, or by being teased with a feather on your ribs. Get to know your own body and what turns you on, whether it's traditional places and moves or unusual ones. Know that sex involves your mind (what you think), your emotions (what you feel), your body image (how you perceive yourself), your body's actions (what you do), your energy (how much energy you have to be sexual and how you

> move your energies within your body and between your body and your partner's), and your spirit (the essence of you).
>
> —Dr. Patti Britton, clinical sexologist

<u>All the Single Ladies . . .</u>

When I first started dating as a single mom, I was filled with insecurities. I was embarrassed and sometimes afraid to mention that I had a child. But the truth is, my son is one of the greatest things about me. If I was patient before, I am even more patient now. If I was giving before, I have much more to give now. And if I was loving before, I have a much larger capacity in my heart for love now. I no longer apologize for being a mom. In fact, it's the first thing I tell someone new. I have never been more proud or more excited about being a mom.

There is no doubt that dating as a single mother has its challenges. Not every man can or wants to step into that kind of relationship. And that's okay. The way I see it, it takes a special man to date a mom, and I know I deserve a special man. My son is my insurance that I end up with someone amazing. So go out there with a healthy sense of self and with confidence about all you have to offer and all that you and your kids deserve. Don't settle. When you have kids, it's critical to have good people around; your partner is a role model who will affect your child's life tremendously. Keep your standards high, for yourself and for your kids. Like attracts like, and in no time, you are sure to attract exactly what you are looking for. Really know and believe that. You are a Hot Mom, after all.

Dating for Two

You heard the phrase "eating for two" when you were pregnant. Dating as a single mom is kind of like *dating for two*: You have to consider how your actions affect your kids. Your priorities change. It is important to find someone who is good to your children, not just good in bed. And if you can find both, wonderful!

A challenge to dating when you have kids is finding the time to actually do so. You have diapers to change and science projects to supervise, you have bedtime books to read and teeth to brush. The key to finding the time to date: Be lucky enough to have joint custody. This way, you have the luxury of having a couple of nights a week free while knowing that your kids are well taken care of.
—Joanne Kimes, author of *Dating Sucks*

One of my favorite comedies about being a single parent is *About a Boy*, starring Hugh Grant. If you haven't seen it, rent it!

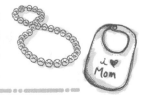

HERE ARE SOME THINGS NOT TO DO AS A SINGLE MOM.

🌼 Act like a teenager. I get it: It's been a while since you dated, and you may be tempted to relive the party days of your youth—or feel like you need to get married so badly that you date every guy who asks you out, in hopes that he just might be "the one."

🌼 Tie your date's shoe. (I actually did that once—it was an unconscious reaction.)

🌼 Introduce your kids to your date too soon. If they hit if off, imagine the disappointment if things go south. Breakups are so much more complicated when there are more hearts involved.

🌼 Talk about how crazy it is that, even though you're finished breastfeeding, your breasts still leak every time you hear a baby cry.

🌼 Refer to yourself in the third person by saying things like, "Don't worry, Mommy is going to make it feel all better"—unless, of course, he asks you to!

🌼 Get discouraged. There are a lot of frogs out there, but there are a lot of princes, too!

Dating Dads

The dating pool has opened up a whole new set of options, including the single dad. Before kids, you probably would not have been open to dating someone with children. Now you realize that dads get it. They get your lifestyle; they understand when the sitter cancels at the last minute or when little Johnny has a seismic meltdown because the ice cream shop is out of Oreo topping. They're less selfish and more patient than men without kids. I personally prefer dating dads. It may be weird to say, but it's a more of a turn-on for me to see a guy in his BabyBjörn—or coaching the soccer team, or just generally being a terrific father to his child—than in his business suit. I have found that a lot of single dads feel the same way about single moms like you.

Keep in mind that some of Hollywood's biggest stars married single moms. Ashton Kutcher married Demi Moore, a mom of three; Matt Damon's wife has a little girl from a previous relationship; Brad Pitt is partnered with the infamous single mom Angelina Jolie; and Seal actually started dating Heidi Klum when she was pregnant!

Whether you are dating or married, one of the great priorities in life—and the ultimate aphrodisiac—is having fun. It's what keeps relationships together.

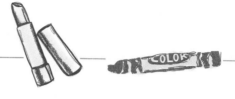

Eight

Blondes Moms Have More Fun!

*With four young children to guide through life, I have made it
my lifelong promise to myself and to my children to be forever
their encourager, to embrace their creativity, and to fill their
lives with all the love their hearts can hold.*

—Holly Robinson Peete, actress, talk show host,
and founder of the HollyRod Foundation

Love your kids; love your life. Duh, right? You'd be surprised
how many moms are so lost in the *Groundhog Day* routine
that they forget to really enjoy the
moment. I was one of them. Years
ago, I was out with Gabe, my five-
year-old, running a laundry list of
errands during a rainstorm. We
were sprinting from the car to the
store and back again, trying des-
perately not to get wet. Anytime he was tempted by a puddle,
I'd instinctively pull him back, telling him to watch his shoes
or his pants.

> "Enthusiasm" comes
> from the Greek word
> entheos, meaning
> "filled with the divine."

At the next stop on my to-do list, I saw a mother carefully

navigating her child around the puddles, the same way I had been. It made me pause and think, "When did I get so responsible?" I tossed my purse in the car, grabbed my son's hand, and stomped right into a puddle, creating a huge splash. He laughed, impressed, and shot me the "Sure it's okay?" look. I nodded, and I can't describe to you the look of joy on his face as he tore into that first muddy puddle of water.

We jumped and laughed. We pounded those puddles and splashed till we were soaked! It was so much fun, such a tremendous release. For those ten minutes, I didn't give an ounce of attention to what I had to do or where I had to go. I was completely wrapped up in living that moment, living that excitement, with him.

> There's no greater love on this planet than that of a mother for her child . . . except maybe fresh funnel cake or a deep-tissue massage, but that's up for debate.
>
> —Joanne Kimes, author of *The Stay-at-Home Martyr*

So I didn't get to the dry cleaners, or the bank, or the post office. In fact, I had to add getting the car washed to the to-do list, as well as an extra load of laundry. But as I tucked my son into bed and told him how much fun I'd had with him, he looked at me with such love and said, "I hope it rains tomorrow, Mom, so *you* can jump in the puddles again."

It's not always practical, but every once in a while, we have to let love pull us into the moment. Let the moment be bigger than the errands on our lists. It's easy to forget, but every moment is an opportunity to create a lasting memory for our children.

Motherhood has, ironically, slowed me down. Everyone catches herself worrying about doing everything right, looking good, being successful at her career—the list goes on. It all seems like a big race sometimes, but to where and for what I'm not too sure. But then I catch a smile on my daughter's face. You know the kind: She just stares at you and suddenly the moment stands still. It is in these moments that we realize we all have this intrinsic ability to be amazed and contented with the world—just as our children do—if we just get ourselves to slow down.

—Jen Mahoney, Hot Mom of two
(and my best friend from college!)

Think about all the blessings in your life and smile. Right now: Smile! Do it. Your children should always remember you smiling. Enjoy your life, no matter how hectic it is; try to remember that every minute is precious and fleeting. Attitudes are contagious. In the midst of the madness, smile. Trust me, it changes everything. Don't take life—or this book—too seriously. Lighten up, be silly. Hot moms are silly and confident. I can think of no better example to set for your kids.

Choose to be happy, and let your face show it. And, yes, it is a choice! If you have been following the other tips in this book, then smiling should come naturally. Remember, you are never more beautiful than when you smile. Create a lasting presence. Shine; a smile can light a room. There is power and magic in a smile. One of my favorite things is my son's smile the minute he sees me after school—and if his smile affects me that much, I can only imagine the effect my smile has on him. Make smiling a habit. Smile at your children playing, smile at those teenagers that can't keep their hands off each other, smile because you still feel that way about your partner, smile at the construction workers who are checking you out, smile because you are well over the drinking age and you still get carded. Smile when your son throws up in your bed—because it had to be the day you washed your sheets! Smile when someone asks if you are the babysitter. Smile when you reply, "No, and I have one more at home twice his age!" Guard your sense of humor with your life!

All day today, smile, no matter what the circumstances—whether your son spills juice in your newly clean car or burps at the table, smile! Remember: The more you smile, the more they will smile. Never underestimate the power of a smile. I have defused many tense situations with a wholehearted smile. Your attitude is contagious, and it affects everything and everyone around you. So, what's that word again? Oh, yeah: SMILE!

Eye contact is a great way to show your strength, your sincerity, and your love. As Tyra Banks says on *America's Next Top Model,* "Smile with your eyes."

One ordinary day, while I was getting the kids dressed to go somewhere, packing the diaper bag, buckling them in the car, and thinking of a hundred different things, my five-year-old son asked me a question. Busy, I replied with a short "I don't know," to which he said, "But, Mommy, you know EVERY-THING." It was as if a ray of light had burst out of the sky and shined down on me, THE ALL-KNOWING ONE! I had to laugh. I smiled and said, "You're right—I *do* know everything." We can't ruin our children's perception of us, now can we?

—Joy Bergin,
cofounder of the Hot Moms Club

Lighten Up and Be Silly!

Hot Moms are in touch with that silly side of them. Sing in the shower; blast a little Lady Gaga and belt out some tunes in the car. Sing, sing, sing with your kids, sing loud, sing off key. Be firm when you need to be firm, and be in charge, but be sure your kids see the lighter side of you. Once a week, my son and I dance. I throw on a fun CD and we get totally goofy: We jump around; I do funny dance moves, he imitates; he busts a crazy move and I copy it. Inhibitions are not part of this moment. We laugh and laugh. By being free, living each second, enjoying the music without inhibitions, you will build your children's confidence and help them to laugh at themselves. Make this a treat, but be sure to make it happen. As much joy as it brings them, it will fill your spirit even more.

We have a nighttime bath ritual that began spontaneously one night. It may sound silly to some people, but for us it is such a blast. Each night, just before the kids get in the tub, we jump on the bed and do a quick round of Ring Around the Rosie—very cutely named "Naked Ashes" by my four-year-old daughter. The kids think it is so cool that they are allowed to hop on our bed naked, and it is always so endearing and wonderful to see my husband enthusiastically participating, with his full business suit still on from work. The kids look forward to this every night, and I want to cherish it as long as I can before they get too big; these are memories and moments I will forever savor.

—Amanda Stephens,
Hot Moms Club member and mom of two

Dance, Dance, Dance

From soft music in the nursery to dance parties, involvement in music strengthens children's educational, physical, and emotional development—plus it gives kids a chance to really let loose and express themselves. Hip-hop classes for elementary-school kids are all the rage, and babies in diapers jamming out to Beyoncé have become a viral Web sensation. And have your ever been to a local Baby Loves Disco event? Let's just say, Donna Summer would be proud. (Go to BabyLovesDisco.com for dates and locations.) From the time we are small, we are inspired to move to rhythms that excite and inspire us.

Music is an essential part of growing up. Child-development researchers can't quite agree on whether exposure to music of particular genres correlates to smarter kids (go ahead—Google "Mozart effect" to see what I mean), but experts do agree that involvement in music strengthens kids' intellectual, physical, and emotional development.

Think about how excited you feel when you hear an old song come on the radio and it transports you back in time. Singing and dancing with your kids regularly will create wonderful memories that will stay with them forever. Kids bond as they take part in fun activities, so now and then, let your hair down, turn the music up, and join your kids. Move to the beat, create fun dance moves, and let your kids see the silly side of you.

Music has the power to connect with everyone. Children respond to all types of musical sounds, and a savvy mom can use music to help control her child's moods. Melodies can energize kids or relax them; fast rhythms can lift up your child's low spirits, and slow, soothing songs can calm restless minds.

Dancing is fun and easy, not to mention great exercise for people of all ages. It gives kids a chance to let loose and express themselves. In a family life packed with activities—and, let's just cop to it, stress—we all could use a little booty shaking. Incorporating music and dance into your daily routine will have an incredible impact on your child's self-esteem and development. Plus, kids love to see their parents act crazy! As a child, you had a rich imagination, so find ways to tap into your creativity again!

HERE ARE SOME OF MY FAVORITE CDS TO ENJOY WITH KIDS.

✿ Meredith Brooks, *If I Could Be . . .*

✿ Barenaked Ladies, *Snack Time*: a fun children's album.

✿ Rhythm Child, *Eat a Bowl of Cherries*: soulful, drum-based music for kids. I have seen Rhythm Child perform, and their energy is off the charts; plus, they really get kids excited and engaged in music.

✿ Putumayo Kids introduces kids to other cultures through music from around the world. The songs are fun; listen to a sample and learn more at Putumayo.com.

✿ For lulling your little one to sleep, the renowned harpist Merry Miller has a collection of beautiful and peaceful CDs to soothe even the fussiest of babies (BabyMusicToGo.com).

Inspiring mom Candi Carter is the creator of It's Hip Hop, Baby!, a series of educational DVDs for children age two to six. Candi's son Emerson suffers from a rare disorder and severe speech delays. In response, Candi became "silly mommy" and started making up songs with hip-hop beats to calm him down during tantrums. It worked. The songs also helped him learn the concepts of words faster. She wondered if these songs could help other children, so she created the series. There are five titles, with more on the way (ItsHipHopBaby.com).

What Did You Call Me?

It's always tricky naming a baby you have never met. When you decide your child's name, it has little to do with them as a person; it based on what you like and don't like. Nicknames tend to work because they are usually given based on personality or an event or

Cougar Town actress Busy Philipps (whose real name is Elizabeth) got her nickname from her parents, because as an infant she was always moving. The nickname stuck and even appears on her driver's license. Having grown up with a nickname her whole life, she decided to officially name her daughter Birdie.

situation. I have no idea when or how I started to call my son Snoosh, but it has become my silly nickname for him and it always makes him laugh. Nicknames are powerful things. With the exception of playground taunts, nicknames tend to bond people. They show a close connection, comfort, and familiarity. If you don't have them already, come up with geeky nicknames for your kids, something special that ONLY YOU can call them. Make up a silly word, something funny or endearing. This is a great idea if you are becoming a stepparent; come up with fun nicknames for your stepkids, something cute tailored to their personalities. It will help them to know that you care.

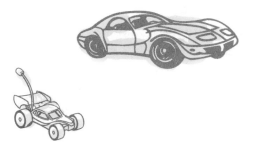

Grow Young!

Your kids are your excuse to stay in touch with the kid inside of you, so swing on the swings with your kids, jump rope, surprise them by sliding down the slide or doing a cannonball into the pool. Start a pillow fight or beep your horn like mad every time you go through a tunnel. Do whatever it is that helps connect a piece of your childhood to theirs.

A Hot Mom is in touch with her silly side and her inner child. Hot Moms know how to have fun. Invite more laughter and playfulness into your life. Be firm with your kids, but be sure to let them see the lighter sillier side of you, too.

Go and run wild with your kids and capture those magic moments that often get lost and neglected due to stress or fatigue. Save the world another day.

—Tracey Mallett, fitness expert

One of the most important things we can give our children and ultimately ourselves as mothers is permission to have adventures. This doesn't have to be anything exotic like cliff diving; to children even the ordinary can be extraordinary.

When my children were young I could have driven them to and from school, but that would have deprived them of the fun of gain-ing some independence and experiencing the change of seasons and puddle jumping! Seeing the look of accomplishment on your child's face when they come home from school after walking in the rain or snow is well worth the cleanup. Hopefully it will bring back memories. So live on the edge. Let your kids play hooky. Go to the beach or take a hike. (They need mental health days, too.) Finger paint with chocolate pudding or lie down in a field and stargaze. By doing fun things, you will connect with your inner children, and your inner child.

—My mom

Curiosity engages us with the surrounding world and keeps our perspective constantly evolving. The act of discovery can be sheer joy. Kids are always learning; don't let your quest for knowledge end when theirs begins.

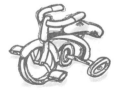

Stop and Smell the Roses

I love flowers, and so does my little girl, Maddy. When she was first learning to walk we would go through the neighborhood picking wildflowers. We would walk and talk about how beautiful they were, what colors they were, their names. Then one day I saw her looking at me curiously every time I would put a flower to my nose. She didn't know what I was doing. So I proceeded to teach her how to "smell the roses." It ain't that easy, folks! The words "inhale" and "exhale" don't have much meaning at this point. For the next few months, every time I would give Maddy a flower she would smile, put it to her nose, and blow snot all over it. Some laughs last forever. Write them down!

—Brooke Burns, actress and
Hot Mom of Maddy

Eat, Cook, Love

Cooking with kids can be so much fun. Letting them help not only occupies them while you are cooking, it helps build their confidence as well as their palates, as they are more apt to try and eat foods if they helped make them. Pizza dough is especially fun to make with kids. They can create their own pizzas, fill calzones, or wrap around hot dogs. I also recommend investing in an ice cream maker, a bread maker, and a pasta maker. Each provides fun activities you can do as a family, and with yummy results.

Can You Dig It?

Plant a garden or grow herbs with your kids. It's fun to watch plants bloom and grow, and your kids will take pride in the fruits and vegetables they produce (and later eat). My son loves to pick limes and lemons from the tree. It is a wonderful way to teach children about connecting with the earth and how everything comes full circle. Go to KidsGardening.org for tips and to order supplies.

When I was growing up, every once in a while my mom would give us a "picnic" dinner on the living room floor. It was same meal we might eat in the dining room, but changing the venue from the table to the floor made it seemed more fun and exciting—and it's funny how the food even tasted better!

HERE'S A LIST OF ONLINE RESOURCES FOR KID-DING AROUND IN THE KITCHEN.

✿ CraftGossip.com has adorable ideas for making art and creatures with food. Click "edible crafts."

❀ FixMeASnack.com is a blog with creative and healthy ideas kids will love,from homemade polka-dot real fruit roll-ups to draw-your-own yogurt (using blackberry sauce, kids "paint" designs in plain yogurt).

❀ JamieOliver.com has great recipes and ideas. Jamie Oliver's TV show *Food Revolution* is great to watch with older kids so they really grasp the concept of healthy eating.

❀ KidsInTheKitchen.org has recipes and ideas to empower kids to make healthy lifestyle choices.

❀ MyDaddyCooks.com is a video blog of dad Nick and his son Archie making all sorts of fun recipes.

❀ Spatulatta.com is a great site devoted to cooking ideas for kids with more than three hundred videos and step-by-step recipes.

❀ Weelicious.com offers a solution to parents' hectic lives by providing recipes that are kid-friendly, quick, and nutritious using few but fresh ingredients.

I wanted my kids to be exposed to new foods and cultures, so each week on Thursday I would make a different dish we had never had before. The rule was, everyone had to try and eat it, and everyone got to rate the dish. If it rated low, I would never make it again, and if it rated high, we could put it into the rotation. Letting the kids and my husband have a say, making them mini food critics, made it a fun game. It made them really think about what they were eating, what they liked and disliked and why, turning trying new things into something to look forward to instead of something to dread. I hope they take that feeling and apply it in all areas of their lives.

—Angela, Hot Mom of three

We have five daughters, so dinner time was getting pretty crazy, with everyone wanting to help and arguing over who was going to sit by Mom or Dad. So, we decided to have the girls take turns helping with dinner. Whoever helped with dinner would also set the dinner table and place the name tags (which the girls designed and created themselves) where she wanted.

Dinner is always a special time when the family makes it a point to sit down and discuss the day. I work as a full time NICU nurse, so juggling work and being a mother is challenging, but this connects us back together every night!

—Lisa Stephens, Hot Mom of five

Think Outside the (Lunch) Box

When it comes to making healthy and appealing school lunches for your kids, you have to be creative but also make it easy on yourself at the same time. Always having a variety of foods on hand that you know your kids love will certainly make it easier to decide what should go in their lunch every day. Focus on healthy items with long shelf lives—dried or dehydrated fruits, certain cheeses, pasta, whole grain breads and crackers, nuts and seeds, nut butters, and frozen vegetables like edamame or broccoli.

I always try to offer balance from the four food groups—fruits and vegetables, some dairy, some protein, and a carbohydrate—so that I know my kids are getting their essential nutritional elements. Also, don't forget that kids are driven not only by the way foods taste, but by the visual aesthetic of what's in their lunch box. When foods are cut into cool shapes or you feature foods with naturally bright colors, the eye appeal alone becomes a huge selling point.

Most important, try and make the entire school lunch experience fun.

Whether you add a dip to make eating more interactive, include a surprise sweet treat that will make your little ones smile, or sneak in a little note, sticker, or toy to brighten their day,

your kids will be excited from the first moment they open their lunch—and hopefully
think of their loving mommy who made it!
—Catherine McCord, founder of
Weelicious.com, alumna of Manhattan's
Institute of Culinary Education,
actress, model, and Hot Mom of two

Start a cooking tree. I know a group of four friends
who divide the week so that each mom is assigned to
a day. Each mom makes five lunches on her day and
sends them to school with her child to give out to the
other moms' kids. They say it is easier to make five
lunches one day a week than one lunch five days.

Match & Munch shaped sandwich cutters (Spoon
Sisters.com, $16.95 for a set of four) make lunchtime
fun.

All through elementary school, my mother
packed my lunch. Every day she wrote a small
note on my napkin. When my daughter, Charlotte, started pre-school at two and a half years
old, I continued the tradition. Every day I made
her lunch, and I included a note wishing her a
great day . . . telling her how proud I was of her,
how much I loved her, etc. One day as I was
leaving her school, her teacher approached me
and told me that they read the notes every day.
The teacher told me how excited Charlotte

> was getting them and how much the other kids also liked hearing them. Charlotte is old enough to read the notes herself now and it still remains one of her favorite things about lunchtime.
>
> —Rob, proud dad of Charlotte

Hot New Product

A Talkatoo is a digital voice recorder that allows you to leave your kids audio messages—for example, saying that you miss them or telling them just how much trouble they will be in if they forget their jacket again. Talkatoos come in a variety of colorful designs that either clip on backpacks or can be worn like a necklace (Talkatoo .com, $16.99).

A Pinch of Fun and a Dash of Wonder

Until you are ready to look foolish, you'll never have the possibility of being great.

—Cher

Whimsy: (n) An odd or fanciful idea.

I am willing to bet we can all benefit from a little more whimsy in our lives. Here are a few small ways you can add a little fun to your mothering.

❀ Skip like a four-year-old. There is nothing like a good skip; I'm smiling right now just thinking about it. Your kids will get a kick out of watching you skip and skipping with you.

❀ Leave secret notes where your kids can find them. Write "I love you" or something that is significant to them on a Post-it note and stash it in their toy box or in their sock drawer. This only takes a second, doesn't cost anything, and is always a welcome surprise.

❀ Keep a few singles in your car's glove box in case you see a kids' lemonade stand. Always try to stop. It never gets old to see the thrill on the kids' faces when they serve you a glass.

❀ Be the mom who has change in her purse for wishing fountains, my son loves this as do I.

❀ Declare backward day. Serve pizza bagels for breakfast and pancakes and eggs for dinner. Or try opposite day and use the opposite words to describe what you are doing. When you pick them up from school, tell them they have to go to a doctor's appointment, but take them for ice cream instead!

❀ Lay on the grass on a cloudy day with the kids and look for shapes in the clouds, or stargaze at night, and set up a tent out in the yard.

❀ Roast s'mores on the stove and camp out in the living room. Make tents, use flashlights, and tell stories.

❀ You never know where the day may take you, so I always keep certain things in the car. We always have towels, a change of clothes, a ball, and a blanket for impromptu trips to the ocean or the park. I also keep an extra sweatshirt for both my son and me in the trunk just in case. We must be prepared for last-minute adventures.

❀ Want to meet your neighbors, or just spread a little cheer? It's simple: Grab your kids, some colorful sidewalk chalk, take a walk in your neighborhood, and write fun and sweet messages by your neighbors' houses like, "Have a great day!" or "I've always wanted to meet you!" This is perfect whether you have moved someplace new or just want to spread some good wishes to old friends.

Plan a Hot Date with Your Kids

Another fun thing you must do as a Hot Mom is to designate a special day (besides his birthday) for just you and your child. I let my son pick a day every year when we go on a "date." It's just for the two of us. It's a priority over anything else. When he was younger I called it Gabe and Mommy Day. He was too young then to really understand the importance of it, but I want him to have as many incredible, magical memories and traditions with me as possible. And it's not just for him; it's for me, too. While our children may outgrow nicknames, your special day can endure. It is never too late to create goofy traditions or memories. This is especially important if you have more than one child. Growing up with a brother and sister, I rarely had my parents' undivided attention, let alone a whole day to spend with one or both of them. Looking back, I would have loved that. Think about the last time you had a magical moment with your child. Now think about when and how you can create one. Make arrangements with each of your kids and plan a day together. Be sure to do something you know they will love—and if you can't carve out a whole day, plan a fun afternoon or evening. Magic is free and limited only by your imagination.

Quality Time

Play Tourist for the Day

Go sightseeing in your own town or a nearby city. When I was growing up in New Jersey, my parents used to take us to New York City often. I've been to the top of the Empire State Building, World Trade Center, and the Statue of Liberty, and I've seen more than my share of shows on Broadway. I was surprised to learn how many of my friends who lived their whole lives only thirty minutes from some of New York City's most famous attractions (some of the most famous attractions in the world) but have never been. We often take things for grated that are right in our figurative backyard. So play tourist and do all the things and see all the sights a tourist would. Take cheesy photographs and collect souvenirs. Your kids will learn about where they live, and who knows, you might learn a cool thing or two, too.

ECO-MINDED MAMA

Bike riding is just plain healthy. It's eco-friendly and a fun way to get in shape while spending time with your kids. This may not be very original, but it is truly one of my favorite activities. It's so freeing and enjoyable, and it's something I wish I did more when my son was small. The truth is, I was afraid I would tip the bike over or not be able to balance, but today there have been many advancements and there are many more options for riding a bike with a little one.

$TUFF TO DROOL OVER

The Taga is a stroller and bike in one (TagaBikes.com, $1,495). It is the only bike that transforms into a stroller. You can use it with newborns, with six-year-olds, with two children at once, or with groceries. It's a favorite of celebrity moms including Kelly Rutherford.

Zigo Leader X1 or X2 Carriers (MyZigo.com, $1,350–$1,399) are stylish and sporty three-wheeled bikes with a zipped "child pod" in the front that carries one or two children easily while you ride.

Buddy Bikes are tandem bicycles (BuddyBike.com, $1,660–$1,880) that are said to be wonderful for kids with special needs who can't right by themselves.

BABY ON A BUDGET

The iBert Safe-T-Seat (iBertInc.com, $95) is a child seat that attaches to the front of your bike and is used by many celebrities including Tori Spelling.

Get Outta Here

Get out of the house! Take your kids to aquariums, zoos, and museums. See what days they offer discounts or free entry. Also, many pet stores have a big selection of fish, hamsters, and interesting animals to look at, and many will let you play with the puppies.

Scope out the local parks in your area and ask around. No matter how fabulous your backyard, kids still love the socialization that a park or playground provides. Some of the custom playgrounds are really amazing, too. When my son was small, we would frequent a park around the corner from us. It was modest, but he loved it. Then I found out through talking with some friends that a brand new playground had been built only five minutes from my house. It was well worth the ride; my son's eyes nearly popped out of his head when he saw all of the play options, which included tunnels and climbing gear.

Get your Hot Moms Club together and make an appointment to bring your kids to the local fire station. It's free, and let's face it, there could be worse things than spending the afternoon with some firemen. Ha!

Scope out a "secret spot" to explore with your kids. Just giving it the name "secret" will make it feel more special and magical. So ask around and see if your friends have secret spots where they take their kids. My friend and her son introduced me to a spot in the canyon not too far from where I live. We found frogs and saw lizards and all sorts of creatures. My son had a blast, and had my friend not showed it to me, I would have never known it was tucked back there. Now it is a favorite little secret spot of ours. You never know what fabulous places are just around the corner.

GoCityKids.com lists fun activities in your area. Just plug in your zip code and search through concerts, parades, and dozens of other activities happening near you each day.

Every city has its "it" spot for moms to hang out. In New York it's Citibabes (CitiBabes.com), or Kidville (Kidville.com). (Kidville is also expanding nationwide.) Divalysscious Moms, also in New York City, hosts the most fabulous events for both moms and kids. Sign up for insider Lyss Stern's newsletter and event calendar at DivaMoms.com. Big City Moms (BigCityMoms.com) is another group in New York City that gives events catering to the stroller set.

In Los Angeles, the Tree House Social Club (The TreeHouseSocialClub.com) is the hot spot for events and activities, with a giant indoor tree house in the center. It is a safe bet that on any given day you will see a celebrity mom or their spawn playing here. When

Suri Cruise is in town it is one of her favorite hangout spots.

The Coop (TheCoopLA.com) is another modern play area for trendy moms and hip kids. Julie Bowen hosted a birthday party for her twins at the Coop and Jennifer Garner and Ben Affleck have attended parties with their girls at the space.

In Chicago, Family Grounds Café (FamilyGrounds Cafe.com) is a kid-friendly coffee shop with a big play area. Enjoy a latte and decadent muffin while your kids play with friends completely in view. I absolutely love this place and this concept. A sign at the front counter jokes, "Unattended children will receive an espresso and a free puppy."

Creativity: (n) 1. The ability to transcend traditional ideas, rules, or patterns. 2. Meaningful and original new interpretations.

$TUFF TO DROOL OVER

KidTropolisBuild.com creates incredible custom-built kids' rooms and backyard tree houses. These functional, one-of-a-kind spaces come with a five-figure price tag.

Geek Dad: Awesomely Geeky Projects and Activities for Dads and Kids to Share, by Ken Denmead, is a book that tells you how to build the best slip-and-slide ever, how to create customized comic strips and board games, how to make a working lamp out of Legos and CDs, and many more fun projects. It's a perfect way for the tech-savvy dad to unleash his inner kid.

BABY ON A BUDGET

Winter fun: Tie a rope to rectangular plastic laundry baskets, place a warm blanket in the bottom, and voilá, you have a sled for a toddler. When you are done sledding, place the basket outside the door for wet shoes and boots. Or try snow painting: Fill several spray bottles with water and food coloring and let the kids go out and create. (I am sure there is a really creative joke about yellow snow that I should insert right here, but I think I'll just let it go.)

Summer fun: Use those same spray bottles for fun water fights that won't kill your water bill like a hose fight does.

ECO-MINDED MAMA

Make bird seed snow angels. Buy bags of different types and different colors of bird seed. Have your child make a snow angel, carefully help him up, then let him decorate the angel with the bird seed. You can use pine boughs as the angel's wings and add pine cones, twigs, and other objects to the design, too.

Sometimes the things we are ready to toss out as trash can be used to entertain our children. I can still vividly remember playing with the old stove boxes and refrigerator boxes in our backyard, rolling and pushing my brother and sister down the hill in the box. It was a blast. Create forts like you did when you were a kid. Let your children make things out of moving boxes.

Make wave boxes. Put a handful of beads in an empty cereal box, then use strong tape to secure the box shut. Rock the box; it will make the sound of waves.

Wash out old yogurt containers, place the lid from a baby food jar inside, seal, and shake.

Place noise-making objects in empty plastic water bottles, make sure the cap is twisted tight and sealed with tape, then let your baby enjoy.

UnpluggedOnARug.com creates "green" play dates, classes, and activities for kids.

Teaching Your Kids Earth-Friendly Living Is as Important as Good Manners

Recycling can be fun and rewarding. When you teach your children to make the connections between nature and the things they use every day, you give them the gift of understanding the importance of protecting the environment—their home. When a child feels useful and does responsible things that have meaning, it brightens his day and boosts his self-esteem. Recycling is mandatory in many communities; why not make it a fun activity for your kids? Set up a recycling center in your home with a couple of bins for sorting materials. Allow your child to decorate and label each bin and he or she can be the recycling captain in your home, making sure the family is separating items properly and rinsing out bottles and cans; or keep score while your child throws the items into the bins (like baskets in a basketball game). Children can also learn about earning and saving money or rewards through recycling. Every time a child disposes of his garbage in the correct recycling bin, affix a sticker to a sticker chart. When a designated number of stickers is collected, offer a reward, such as a small toy or favorite treat. Or get your children to help collect bottles and cans and return them to a recycling center, and teach them to save and budget the money they receive. The more cans they collect, the more money they will receive—now, that's green incentive. No matter how big or small your children are, when they watch you recycle and take care of the planet, you set a good example and show them how much you care for them, and our Mother Earth.

—Beth Aldrich, green living expert and Hot Mom of three

For more information on recycling, visit Recycle Bank.com or BottlesAndCans.com.

Pirates of the Dodge Caravan

Because my parents live on the opposite coast, my son has been traveling on airplanes since he was two months old to visit his grandparents. Like his mom, he loves to travel. Today, I travel for work and pleasure. Not a month goes by that I am not on at least one flight. I know many moms who are paralyzed by the thought of traveling with their kids, be it by car or by plane. As someone who has traveled alone with a child from the

> *There is no such thing as fun for the whole family.*
> —Jerry Seinfeld

time he was an infant, I feel I can tell you: Just do it. If you are prepared, you will be fine. So I encourage you to plan a fun trip for the family this year, be it a road trip or someplace by plane. Do something different. Go somewhere you have never been before. Get brave! Have an adventure!

Natalie Klein, Hot Moms Club products editor and travel writer for *Mom* magazine, and I have pulled together a list of some of our favorite tips and products to make traveling with little ones a heck of lot easier:

As soon as your child is old enough to walk by herself, get her a rolling backpack to bring on the plane. I let her pack it with the toys and snacks she likes.

For very young children, buy several inexpensive small toys (one for each thirty minutes of travel) and wrap them as little presents. The unwrapping will keep them occupied for as long as the toys will, and you can bring a new one out when they get bored.

I have never tried this, but one of our members says that a ball of sticky masking tape will occupy a toddler on a flight for long time.

If you don't have time to pull together a bunch of the games your child likes, TravelKiddy.com offers prepacked travel activities designed for all age groups. A Velcro strap attaches the bag to a seatbelt to keep it all in place.

MomsMinivan.com is a great resource with more than 101 travel game ideas for road trips.

A Zoobie (Zoobies.com) is a stuffed animal, pillow, and blanket all in one—perfect for sleeping in the car or on an airplane.

The Baby B'Air Flight Vest (BabyBAir.com, $34.95) is one solution to safely flying with a baby on your lap.

You put the vest on your baby and then thread your seatbelt through a loop in the back of the vest. If you hit turbulence, the child will not fall out of your arms. (FAA regulations permit use of this device during flight only, not during takeoff, taxi, or landing.)

Great news! If your child is more than a year old and weighs twenty-two to forty-four pounds, you don't need to lug that cumbersome car seat onto the plane. CARES, which stands for the Child Aviation Restraint System, is a system of belts for your child's airplane seat that can be used as an alternative to a car seat (available at KidsFlySafe.com for $74.95). It's convenient because it's small and weighs only a pound, so you can throw it in your purse. CARES gives you the added protection that your child will remain stable throughout the flight. If you travel by plane a bit, maybe going back and forth to Grandma's, this may be worth the investment.

The Gogo Kidz Travelmate (GogoBabyz.com, $89.99) significantly lightens the load for parents on the go with babies, toddlers, and all their gear. It's a convenient and safe attachment with wheels, suitable for a variety of car seats, that allows you to roll your child and his car seat through the airport instead of carrying them.

The Sit 'n' Stroll (LillyGold.com, $249.95) is both a car seat and a stroller. You can take it out of your car and turn it into a stroller, wheel it right onto the plane, then change it back to a seat.

Keep your baby's formula cold during a flight. You can pack an insulated bag, then ask the flight attendant for some ice, or you can chill the bottle by filling the air-sickness bag with ice and putting the bottle right in there. It'll keep it cold for a long time and will be ready whenever your baby wakes up. It's like having your own mini-fridge.

When traveling with infants and small children, you are allowed to pre-board, and there are also often special security lines or fast-track customs check points for people traveling with small children.

A couple of great online resources are TravelWith YourKids.com, which has tips on—you guessed it—traveling more easily with your kids, and WeJustGot Back.com has reviews of kid-friendly hotels, advice from families who have been there, and lots of deals and ideas.

BABY ON A BUDGET

Most people like to plan their vacations well in advance to be sure they get the exact accommodations they want and what they think is the best deal—but last-minute vacations can be a great way to find incredible bargains. Some of the best hotels offer great rates on last-minute reservations when their occupancy is low. If you can be flexible, these sites have amazing steals for a last minute jaunt or a quick vacation:

✿ FamilyGetaway.com

✿ Hotels.com

✿ LastMinute.com

❁ Buddy Fruits are like smoothies to go, packaged in a small pouch that can easily be
tossed out (BuddyFruits.com).

❁ Clif Kid's Organic ZBars are low in fat with whole
oats and twelve essential vitamins and miner-
als. They come in a variety of yummy flavors like
honey graham and chocolate brownie. Clif Kid
Organic Twisted Fruit Snacks are also delicious and
contain one serving of fruit each. Both products
are available at ClifBar.com.

❁ Gerber.com (Yogurt melts, bring the calcium
without the mess of yogurt).

❁ Little Duck Organics are a dehydrated fruit
snacks that taste like candy. (Go to Little
DuckOrganics.com for retailers.)

❁ Popchips are my son's favorite and a go-to treat
for when we travel (Popchips.com for retailers).

Traditions

Traditions are said to be the glue that binds a family
together through the generations. What traditions are
you carrying on, and what traditions are you starting
with your kids? Here are some ideas.

School Year's Eve?

The start of the school year is like the kids' New Year. They get a new class, a fresh start. With summer coming to a close, it can be a tough transition. Hot Moms can make sure they kick off the school year right.

Every year on the first day of school, my parents would make us take a picture in our front yard in the same spot. We hemmed and hawed and complained, but I am so happy we did it. I love looking back on those photos and seeing how much we had grown from year to year, how much the background changed as well, and our choice of outfits. Taking the photo in the same spot really gives a good context and makes the changes that much more apparent. So when your kids are heading off to school, start a photo tradition. Be consistent, and no matter how much they complain, make it happen. Everyone will thank you later.

I have heard of moms who have had their kids hold up a sign that says something like "Starting 1st Grade" or simply the number of the grade they were entering.

One mom I know planted a tree when her daughter entered kindergarten. She plans to take a photo by the tree every year. What a great way to show the passage of time.

I always a make a special dessert the first day of school, something over the top that helps my son celebrate the start of his new year and puts him in the frame of mind that it will be fun and exciting.

New Year's Eve

New Year's doesn't have to be a tough holiday to celebrate with kids. When the kids are small, a great way to include them in the celebration is to turn the clocks ahead. It is New Year's Eve somewhere in the world; pick a country and celebrate when they do. I live on the West Coast, and we always celebrate with New York City, so the kids are in bed early and then the adults can enjoy!

BABY ON A BUDGET

Most of the excitement of New Year's is watching your kids let loose. Save bubble wrap from your holiday gifts, and as your countdown begins, have the kids get ready to stomp on it all at once when you get to zero. It sounds just like firecrackers. You can also take the celebration out to your driveway. This is always a big hit. (It is also a safe alternative to firecrackers for Fourth of July parties.)

Let kids decorate cardboard paper towel and toilet paper rolls with markers and stickers, glue streamers on the ends, tape a long stick to the inside so it is easy to hold, then they can wave it like a flag.

Cheers!

My son loves to clink glasses and say "cheers." Make Shirley Temples (add a dash of grenadine to ginger ale and top with a cherry) and be sure to pick up some colorful fancy (plastic) glasses to make it seem special. You can also let your kids decorate a personal New Year's Eve cup, describing in one word or phrase their feelings about the year or predictions for the next under the date. Use the same cup each year and update it; as the kids grow, it will be fun to read their thoughts from the year before. (Target, Walmart, and most craft or dollar stores have all the supplies you need for designing your own New Year's cup.)

Fortune Cupcakes?

Part of the excitement of the New Year is wondering and hoping about all there is to come and what the future may hold. Make a batch of cupcakes for your family or guests. Before you frost them, cut index cards in quarters or pieces small enough to fit in the cupcakes and write fortunes on each. You can keep them all generic, or personalize them for each family member specifically—so if you have a sister who is pregnant, hers might say, "I see many sleepless nights" or "I see triplets in your future"; your husband's might say, "Pampering your wife will lead to just rewards." You know your guests, so be creative. Once your fortunes are written, punch a hole in each tiny card, tie curling ribbon through, and wrap it tightly in tin foil. Insert each fortune into a cupcake (making a slit with a sharp knife might make this easier) and frost them so that only the ribbons are sticking out. When you serve them, have everyone pull their ribbons and read their fortunes.

Holidays

Family and tradition are what the holidays are all about, right?

My mom used to host a holiday cookie exchange for all the moms on our street each year just before the holidays. Each mom had to bring two dozen of their favorite type of holiday cookie and an extra plate. The moms would fill their empty plates with a sample of all the other moms' homemade cookies so they would have a good mix to take home for out-of-town guests and their families. Not only did this save them all the work of baking so many kinds, but it was a fun night of socializing, too.

Jingle Bells

Let the kids make jingle bell bracelets. All you need is a pack of pipe cleaners, some jingle bells, and some colorful beads. These can be worn on ankles as well as wrists. Kids can also make them for family members and party guests. This will not only be fun but keep them busy.

> As a kindergarten teacher, Ryan's mom loved reading her students a book called *Alfie the Christmas Tree*, by John Denver, during the holidays. It is not only her favorite book during the season, but one of ours as

well . . . especially now that we have babies! The book's basic message is to celebrate the beauty of nature, so each year, we "decorate" pine cones with peanut butter and bird seed and hike up through the gorgeous mountains of Vail, Colorado, to a tree that we have designated as our very own "Alfie." In my mind, it is a great way to spend quality time with our family and also teach our kids to appreciate the beauty of the world we live in and the scenic backyard we call home.

—Trista Sutter, proud mommy of Max and
Blakesley and (to most everyone else)
The (original) Bachelorette

Thanksgiving

A friend of mine's mom has a keepsake tablecloth she displays every Thanksgiving. It includes baby hand- or footprints and little notes and signatures from guests of all of her feasts. My friends says it brings tears to eyes when she reads the notes from her beloved grandfather and when she looks at the clumsily written messages she and her siblings wrote when they were small. Now her kids' handprints are on this very special tablecloth. It may not be fancy, but it has so much meaning and each year reminds her what being thankful is all about.

Guess the Cranberries

Fill a beautiful jar with cranberries and set it on the table. This doubles as a gorgeous centerpiece. Throughout the meal let everyone guess how many cranberries they think are inside. After the meal, count, and make sure you have a good prize for the person who guessed closest!

The Gratitude Box

Let the kids decorate an old shoe box. Cut a whole in the top and set it out with pieces of paper and pencils and pens. When your guests arrive, have each write down two or three things they are grateful for—but without signing their names. Make sure everyone drops their thoughts into the box. At dinner, open the box and start reading. Everyone will have fun guessing who said what. This activity often leads to touching discussions.

Halloween

Roasting pumpkin seeds is one of my favorite Halloween traditions. Clean the seeds you scooped from your pumpkins when you carved them. Spread the seeds on a cookie sheet, add melted butter, some brown sugar, and salt to taste. Bake for forty-five minutes, stirring occasionally. Cool and enjoy.

Go pumpkin picking! This year, visit an authentic pumpkin patch. Walking between the pumpkin rows until you find the perfect pumpkin is truly an experience for adults and children alike. Search for farms within driving distance from your home. It is well worth the trip. Many farmers will take you on a tractor ride to the pumpkin patch.

Have you ever tasted fresh apple cider? If your answer is no, then you need to put this book down and find an orchard near you. This is one of the things I miss most about growing up on the East Coast, along with fall leaves and going apple picking. There is nothing like the taste of fresh apple cider in the fall. Apple picking is also a lot of fun. It is the perfect fall family adventure.

Celebrate

Whether it's using a special birthday plate or customizing a scavenger hunt to find gifts, birthdays are the perfect time for personal traditions that make the kids feel special.

We have a special birthday song that my mother sang to us every year and that her mother sang to her. Not a birthday has gone by that I haven't also sung this song to my kids. The lyrics are simple and it leads you right in to the "Happy Birthday" song.

So today is your birthday, that's what I've been told,
What a wonderful birthday you are now [X] years old.
On the cake there are candles all lighted for you

*And the whole world is singing
"Happy Birthday to You."*

There is a pause and then everyone sings "Happy Birthday."

—Joy Bergin,
cofounder of the Hot Moms Club

To celebrate birthdays in our house, the kids are treated to breakfast in bed. So from the moment you first peel your eyelids open, you know that the day belongs to you, in all of your uniquely special ways, as your siblings stand at your bedside, with candles stuck in everything from strawberries to muffins, to pancakes and bananas, belting out "Happy Birthday" as you shake the cobwebs out of your brain. And your birthday launches . . . from the minute you wake!

—Robyn O'Brien, founder of AllergyKids Foundation, author, and Hot Mom of four

Let's Party!

The Hot Moms Club has a reputation for throwing lavish and unique celebrity baby showers, first birthday parties, and events that have been featured in *People*, *Us* weekly, *Life & Style*, and *OK!* magazine. Hot Moms

Club's planner Natalie Klein, the Hot Moms Club team, and I have worked with countless celebrities to customize and make their children's event memorable. Below are some of our favorite tips and tricks for creating a birthday party like you see in the magazines, one that is sure to wow your friends and most importantly please your kids. It is more budget-friendly than you would guess. First, find your inspiration or theme, and then go, go, go! With the Internet at your fingertips, you can Google for the best of the best without breaking the bank.

Invitations set the tone for a party. Paper invitations can be fun and a bit more of an expense, but if you plan ahead you can find good deals. Order them online from companies like TinyPrints.com, Shutterfly.com, and NestingShoppe.com. For e-mail invitations, which cost less, try sites like PaperlessPost.com, Evite.com, MyPunchbowl.com, and SmileBox.com. These sites also give you an easy way to manage your guest list.

I actually received a video invitation recently, by e-mail. A friend's adorable son was inviting my son to his party, and the video showed him reciting (with the help of his parents) all of the details. I thought this was really clever. If you do this be sure to follow up with a paper invitation for those people who can't download the video or for guests who might not be Web savvy. If you don't have a video camera, the very affordable Flip video recorder (TheFlip.com, $149.99–$249.99) is perfect for this. It's sleek and fits into any purse or pocket. And it comes with HD options that would make Spielberg proud.

Décor

Décor should be fun but reusable. Some of our favorite websites to visit for inspiration and themes are HostessWithTheMostess.com, Momologie.com, Tom KatStudio.blogspot.com, and MarthaStewart.com/kids.

Set the table with personalized plates and items for your guests. EmTannerDesigns.com is a good source.

"Presents" make a fun and affordable centerpieces. Find beautiful wrapping paper and ribbon that coordinates with your theme, wrap boxes of different sizes, and place them next to one another on the table. You can even place little presents in them for the guests to take home. If you choose to leave them empty, leave the bottom undone so you can fill them up with a present later on and reuse.

Fill small clear vases and jars with candy for a pop of color (jelly beans work really well). Have a scooper close by, and when the party is over send the guests home with candy bags tied with a pretty ribbon. To purchase candy in bulk go to SweetFactory.com or ACandyStore.com.

Decorated frames with the pictures of the birthday boy or girl always make for a charming centerpiece.

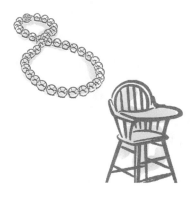

Become the Goddess of Something!

Leave an imprint, personalize the way you entertain. We all possess creative skills and we tend to ignore the fabulousness under our noses. Become the "Goddess" of something. It doesn't matter what, just make it your own—your signature. Declare yourself the goddess of chocolate, or of homemade lasagna, this summer I was the goddess of the "Pool Party"—always hosting my daughter's friends.

—Allana Baroni, Hot Mom, author,
and founder of GetSocial.com

Crowd Pleasers

With kids especially it is important to always have a "snack-tivity." Here are some food options that are guaranteed to make your party stand out.

French Fry Bar

Use both sweet potatoes and regular potatoes. Sprinkle different seasonings on the potatoes when you cook them to give kids a variety of options—cinnamon, sugar, garlic, and seasoned salt, to name a few. Set up the fries in little containers and have plenty of dips, like ketchup, barbeque sauce, honey mustard, mayonnaise, etc. Both the kids and the grown-ups will love this!

To make the french fries, wash regular and sweet potatoes, cut into slices, then cut again to make large matchstick shapes. Put the potatoes into a mixing bowl and toss in some olive oil. Make sure all of the fries are coated, then add your various seasonings as you put them on a baking sheet covered with nonstick spray. Bake for ten minutes. Flip the fries with a spatula, then bake for another ten minutes until done. Cool a few minutes and serve.

Chocolate Tasting Bar

Tasting chocolate is different from eating chocolate. The fun is in making sure you have a selection of different types of chocolates and unusual flavors. Break them into squares and let guests sample them. Pair them with interesting dips, like peanut butter, fruit jams, whipped cream, fudge, and wine. Talk to a chocolate shop owner for suggestions. Some companies will even come and create a chocolate tasting bar for you.

VosgesChocolate.com has many interesting chocolate flavors—including bacon chocolate!

Mashed Potato Martinis

This is a crowd pleaser and easy to make. (Everything just feels more fun served in a martini glass!)

What you need:

Plastic martini glasses in fun colors (available at Target .com or a party supply store)

Potatoes
Chives
Cheddar cheese
Sour cream (or Greek strained yogurt)
Chopped bacon
Avocado
Shredded carrots
Chopped tomatoes
Chopped chicken

Mash your potatoes to your liking then set them out in a large bowl, with all the fixings in little bowls. Let kids create their own custom "martinis" with the mashed potatoes and toppings.

For adults, you can use real martini glasses, add some wasabi to the mashed potatoes, and then serve with shrimp.

Pizza Pizza

This is another really simple crowd pleaser. Have an Italian-themed night with friends. Grab some gourmet pizzas from Trader Joe's (usually around $3–$4 apiece). Then add veggie and meat toppings and drizzle some extra-virgin olive oil on top. This can turn a modest pie into something that looks like it came from a restaurant. Letting kids create their own pizzas and toppings is always fun, too. You can buy pre-made plain pizzas or make them from scratch.

Desserts

Make a batch of cupcakes with a special one for the birthday boy or girl, but leave the others plain—not even frosted. Fill up bowls of frosting and sprinkles and have a contest to see who can make the most creative cupcake. Not only will this take up some time but you won't have anyone upset that they did not get the cupcake they want. This can also be done with a sheet cake.

What to Do About the Swag

Finding party favors that everyone loves can be tough. Reusable treat bags can be personalized and they will be used again and again. Purchase canvas candy bags, give the kids clothing markers, and let them decorate their own.

Mabel's Labels (Mabel.ca) is a good source for personalized gift bags and other items.

Fake tattoos, ChapSticks, and flower seed packets for planting are all affordable and practical trinkets to fill treat bags.

These websites that have adorable party favors and ideas: PlumParty.com, Beau-Coup.com, Oriental Trading.com, BirthdayInABox.com.

Only Hearts Pets (OnlyHeartsClub.com) are small collectable stuffed animals that both young boys and girls will like. They come on a removable keychain that lets kids secure them to their backpacks or belt loops.

Scrapbooking has become more and more popular.

Adding a scrapbooking station to a birthday party is a great way to get relatives involved, not to mention that it helps distribute the work! Check out ShopSEI.com for products and ideas.

Become the Mama-razzi

You are experiencing some of the most exciting times of your life during the early years of motherhood. You are creating so many memories with your little ones; record them in any and every way that you possibly can. You will never regret having those videos, journals, photos, or blogs. Have a journal just for the funny things your kids say. You think you will remember them without writing them down, but trust me, you won't. One of your best investments is a good camera, as well as a small digital one that fits easily into your purse or diaper bag. Be sure to actually get in the photos yourself. My son's baby albums are filled with him and his dad, and once when we were looking through it he asked me, "Mom, where were you?" I said, "Who do think was taking the pictures?" Make sure you jump in some shots too now and then. (For fun visit AwkwardFamilyPhotos.com.)

Photo books have become the new scrapbook. It doesn't matter if you have the crafting skills of a sumo wrestler; you can create a photo book online. You just upload your pictures, write your captions, and choose the backgrounds. It's so easy, even I can do it (and I have).

Nancy O'Dell, a mom, former *Access Hollywood* co-anchor, and admitted scrapbook addict, has a collection with Creative Memories and a book for scrappers called *Full of Love*. Nancy shares a few tips for super scrapping:

1. Use your own handwriting. People often worry that theirs isn't neat enough, but I love seeing my mother's and grandmother's handwriting in old albums; their writing is a memory, too.

2. Write more than your typical captions—but they don't have to be a journal entry! For instance, under my stepson's graduation picture with his baby sister, I wrote, "Ashby was so excited for Tyler that during the whole ceremony she kept yelling, 'Hey, Ty Ty!'"

3. Photograph the not-so-obvious memories: your toddler's precious curls on the back of his head, close up; your daughter's favorite dress; shoes in a pile near the front door.

4. Just get started! Don't fret if you have a box full of photos somewhere from years ago. You don't want to miss out on memories that are happening right now because you feel you have to catch up first. You'll eventually get to that box.

This year for my daughter's eleventh birthday I made an album of the last ten years of her life. I put her photographs with Santa and every year on her birthday side by side so you could really see how she grew and changed throughout the years. She loved it.

—Chris O'Donnell, actor and dad of five

Blogging Is the New Black

Blogging wasn't even a word when my son was born. But blogging the baby is all the rage now. Heck, kids with baby teeth have Twitter accounts and websites. Family websites are especially great if your relatives are all over the country. You can upload photos for everyone to see. TheFamilyPost.com, FamilyCrossings.com, and MyFamily.com are a few websites that allow you to create a family page to post videos, photos, and message boards for your invited family and friends to privately view.

Fun-damentals

*HERE ARE A FEW LITTLE THINGS
THAT MAKE ME AND MY SON HAPPY.*

❀ The ABC comedy *Modern Family* makes
me laugh out loud every episode. It is real.
The characters are well thought out and
hilarious. If you miss the show on TV you can
catch full episodes for free at CastTV.com or
Hulu.com.

❀ My son loves animals, so his guilty pleasure
is a website called DailySquee.com. It has
all the cute little critters you can handle on
one site.

❀ Uno is a classic. This game has entertained
my son for hours—literally. We have been
trapped on many a cross-country flight and
I'm pretty sure we have set world records for
the most consecutive Uno games. It's also a
great family game. Spoons is another classic
that is fun when you have a big family.

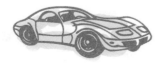

Aim to Create
Endless Perfect Little Moments

The world will never be perfect, and your home will never be perfect (so let it go), but you CAN carve out perfect moments—and lots of them. Make FUN your mantra, and make sure that your children have a packed lifetime of memories with you. Your relationship with your children is the first one they have and it will set the foundation for all of their future relationships. So no matter what your personal obstacles are or how many hours you must work in a day to get by, find time to talk to your kids, teach your kids, and just be with your kids. That really is the fun part. The world is filled with treasures; we have to open ourselves and our children up to all of the wonder that surrounds us daily. Take it all in. Treasure everything. You will never be the perfect mom, nor will I, nor will anyone, BUT you are a Hot Mom, so shine your light bright and enjoy these times—*right now!*

> *If the world was perfect, it wouldn't be.*
> —Yogi Berra

> *The country clubs, the cars, the boats— your assets may be ample, But the best inheritance you can leave your kids is to be a good example.*
> —Barry Spilchuk

Acknowledgments

Where Credit Is Due!

Thank you, thank you, thank you, to all of the amazing mothers and women who contributed their stories and ideas to this book. I am so fortunate to know some of the funniest and most talented bloggers and writers in the business. A special shout out to Minsun Park, Stefanie Wilder-Taylor, Kristen Chase, and Joanne Kimes for their contributions. Thank you also to the talented actress Lauren Holly for writing the Foreword and giving everyone a peek at her life as a mom of three boys. You all define a Hot Mom inside and out.

There are so many people who have supported this book and the Hot Moms Club: Rebekah Whitlock—I will be forever grateful to you for getting the ball rolling and giving me my first chance as an author. Claire Gerus, my super agent, for finding the series a new home at HarperCollins—I couldn't be happier. A HUGE thank-you to May Chen, Amanda Bergeron, Kendra Newton, and the entire HarperCollins team for your patience and devotion to making this series a success.

A million thanks to the Hot Moms Club team. Without your belief in me and your dedication to the brand, this book would not be possible. My deepest gratitude to Joy Bergin, Natalie Klein, Michelle Fryer, Jeff Federman, Greg Klein, Tom Mazza, Maggie, Keri Boyd, Steve Brown, Kirsten Mangers, Jennie Goodwin, GG Benitez, Jeff Von Lom, Julie and Bob Stein, Larry Brandt, Ann Noder, and Kathleen Rinehart. I would also like to thank our sister team at *Mom* magazine for their support and promotion of my books and the Hot Moms Club brand. Thanks also to Abbie Tuller, Debbie Klett, Robert Hold, and the entire Future US staff.

Thank you to my parents, Jeff and Gail, sister Kim, brother Jeffrey and sister-in-law Jennifer, my son Gabriel, his dad Bryan, Rob, Charlotte, and my goddaughter Alana. Without them I wouldn't have any fun stories to tell, and without their love and encouragement I would never have been able to write this. Thank you. Words cannot describe how lucky I feel to have all of you in my life.

Oprah, Martha Stewart, Mae West, Madonna, Audrey Hepburn, Marianne Williamson, J. K. Rowling, Judge Judy, Hillary Clinton, Jane Goodall, Shakti Gawain, Diane von Furstenberg, Rachael Ray, Holly Robinson Peete, Barbara Walters, Tamara Mellon, Angelina Jolie, and Heidi Klum: These are all mentors to me. Some of these women I have had the fortune of meeting; most I have not. They may not know me, but I know them in my heart. They have had a profound impact on my life—they have proved to me that with hard work, focus, and dedication to something you love or passion for what you do, you can succeed no matter what the circumstances. May the world have many more extraordinary women like them.

About the Author

Jessica Denay

Jessica Denay is the founder of the Hot Moms Club, editor at large for *Mom* magazine, and monthly "Mommywood" columnist for *Pregnancy* magazine. As *OK!* magazine's celebrity mom and baby expert, Jessica has her fingers on the pulse of Hollywood mom trends and baby products. She is regarded as a top blogger and mom lifestyle authority, having appeared on more than a hundred television shows, including the *Today* show, *The Tyra Banks Show*, *Entertainment Tonight*, *Access Hollywood*, *E!*, and CNN as well as in dozens of magazines and radio shows giving advice on everything hot for moms. Jessica and the Hot Moms Club have coordinated events, star-studded baby showers, and nurseries for dozens of celebrities including Brooke and Charlie Sheen, Trista Sutter, Alison Sweeney, Jenny McCarthy, Kelly Rutherford, Chandra Wilson, Lauren Holly, and many others. When she's not taking her son to school or the beach, she's busy writing the next installment in the Hot Moms series.

About

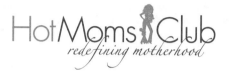

A new Jersey native and former teacher, Jessica Denay along with her friend Joy Bergin created the Hot Moms Club in 2005. It first began as a joke and fun way to boost her own confidence as well as her friends', but the club soon became so popular that Denay was prompted to turn the Hot Moms Club into a business. She credits its success to the timeliness and popularity of the message, "You are not the best mom unless you are the best YOU!" The Hot Moms Club was one of the first websites to speak to moms as women, not just as parents. They define "HOT" as confident and empowered; it doesn't matter what age you are, what shape, or what size, EVERY mom can be a Hot Mom! It's an attitude and way of being. Visit HotMomsClub.com to see what all the hype is about, and join the Hot Moms Club group on Facebook or follow Hot Moms Club on Twitter at HotMomsClubBuzz.

Books by
JESSICA DENAY

The Hot Mom to Be Handbook
Look and Feel Great from Bump to Baby

ISBN 978-0-06-178735-5 (paperback)

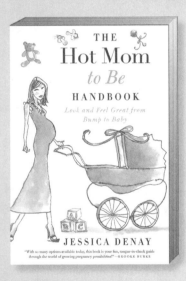

The ultimate resource for any mom-to-be who refuses to check her sense of style and self at the white picket fence.

"The club every mom wants to be a part of."
—Tyra Banks

The Hot Mom's Handbook
Laugh and Feel Great from Play Date to Date Night

ISBN 978-0-06-178737-9 (paperback)

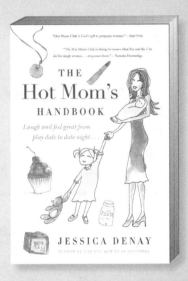

A guide for any Hot Mom who meets the needs of her family but refuses to lose herself in the madness of motherhood.

"There is a new group of mothers that is sweeping the nation—The Hot Moms Club."
—*Today Show*